DATE DUE			

Degradation
of
Chemical
Carcinogens

Degradation
of
Chemical
Carcinogens

An
Annotated Bibliography

M.W. Slein and E.B. Sansone

Environmental Control and Research Laboratory
Frederick Cancer Research Center
Frederick, Maryland

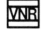 VAN NOSTRAND REINHOLD COMPANY
NEW YORK   CINCINNATI   ATLANTA   DALLAS   SAN FRANCISCO
LONDON   TORONTO   MELBOURNE

Van Nostrand Reinhold Company Regional Offices:
New York   Cincinnati   Atlanta   Dallas   San Francisco

Van Nostrand Reinhold Company International Offices:
London   Toronto   Melbourne

Copyright © 1980 by Litton Educational Publishing, Inc.

Library of Congress Catalog Card Number: 79-19671
ISBN: 0-442-24489-4

Manufactured in the United States of America

Published by Van Nostrand Reinhold Company
135 West 50th Street, New York, N.Y. 10020

Published simultaneously in Canada by Van Nostrand Reinhold Ltd.

15 14 13 12 11 10 9 8 7 6 5 4 3 2 1

Library of Congress Cataloging in Publication Data

Slein, M   W
     Degradation of chemical carcinogens.

     "Research supported by the National Cancer Institute
under contract no. NO1-CO-75380 with Litton Bionetics,
inc."
     Includes index.
     1. Carcinogens—Bibliography. 2. Decomposition
(Chemistry)—Bibliography. 3. Carcinogens—Biodegradation—Bibliography. I. Sansone, Eric Brandfon,
1939-   joint author. II. Title.
Z6664.C2S55 [RC268.6]   016.6148'312   79-19671
ISBN 0-442-24489-4

INTRODUCTION

The substances included in this compilation represent those identified by the U.S. DHEW in 1976 as the organic chemicals for which application of safety standards for research involving chemical carcinogens was to become mandatory. This annotated bibliography was prepared in the hope that it would prove to be useful to persons in small laboratories, as well as to those involved in large-scale production or waste-disposal programs, who must select procedures for the degradation and disposal of chemical carcinogens. Perhaps this compilation will stimulate the development of methods for degrading toxic materials where none is available, or lead to improvements in procedures that already exist.

It should be stressed that few, if any, of the approaches cited have been validated for their efficiency, their safety, or the harmlessness of the resulting products.

Because of space limitations, the tables cannot always include the details presented in the source material. The original sources invariably should be consulted before attempting to apply the procedures described in the tables. It is strongly recommended that the procedures be validated before they are put into use. It is imperative that the procedures be reviewed and approved by the local safety organization before they are implemented.

More often than not, the degradation or reaction products have not been identified and/or their toxicities have not been adequately determined. Degradation products may be even more hazardous than the parent compounds; e.g., diazomethane, which is both explosive and toxic, is formed during the alkaline hydrolysis of some nitroso derivatives. Polychlorinated biphenyls may yield products that are more toxic than the original materials. The lactone rings of aflatoxins can be hydrolyzed by alkali to give less toxic, nonfluorescent substances that are readily reconverted to the fluorescent lactones by subsequent exposure to acids. In other cases, degradation procedures may involve risks other than toxicity, such as the possibility of deflagrations or explosions. Some potential hazards have been identified in the annotations, and one should be aware of them before attempting to apply any procedures for the degradation, decontamination, or disposal of toxic compounds. No attempt was made to indicate specific degradative procedures based on type-reactions for functional groups of the organic compounds in this bibliography other than those which appeared during the literature search.

Information for this bibliography was compiled from various sources, such as the *Merck Index, IARC Monographs,* and *CRC Handbook of Reactive Chemical Hazards,* but the bulk of it was gleaned from some of the data bases available at the library of the Frederick Cancer Research Center. The data bases used were Toxline, Toxback, Chemcon, and Chem 7071. Chemical synonyms and

Chemical Abstract Service (CAS) registry numbers used in the searches were obtained from the computerized Chemline data bank of the National Library of Medicine, as well as from several published sources. Relevant CAS numbers are given after the chemical name in the table headings, and are listed in numerical order at the end of the text. Not all CAS numbers have been included, notably in the case of polychlorinated biphenyls and aflatoxins, which have many structural variants.

It is certain that some relevant references were overlooked—for example, when the data banks searched did not include the descriptor terms in the title, abstract, or key-word list of a stored citation. Older articles may also have been omitted because they were not included in the computerized bibliographies. In many cases, older references were obtained by searching through the bibliographies of publications, beginning with the more recent ones. However, this literature search has not been comprehensive and a further investigation may be made by the reader, using the citations given here as starting points for the retrieval of other references.

Articles concerned with *in vivo* and *in vitro* enzymatically-catalyzed degradation reactions generally have been omitted, since they were considered to be impractical for the resolution of most disposal problems. However, citations dealing with metabolic transformation of toxic compounds by microorganisms, especially as applied to treatment of effluent wastewaters and soil decontamination, have been included because of their actual or potential value. Where the number of publications has been very large, representative examples were selected for inclusion. For example, due to the widespread interest in hydrazine derivatives as rocket propellants, their oxidation has been intensively studied, and many papers on this subject have been published.

An attempt has been made to limit the terminology used in describing degradation techniques in the tables without becoming too nonspecific. With few exceptions, when several reactions for decomposing a substance or group of substances are given in a citation, the general term "chemical" has been used as a descriptor. "Thermal" includes procedures such as cooking, autoclaving, and pyrolzying, but not combustion or incineration, which are included under the term "oxidation." Related procedures are grouped together in the tables as much as possible without repeating any entries that include multiple degradation techniques.* In some cases, no degradation process is given, but an entry has been made to call attention to a special hazard or to an adsorption method which merely removes the material of interest from the gas or solution that it is contaminating.

*To avoid extensive renumbering and retyping of citations and cross-references, relevant citations from monthly updates of the Toxline data base through 1978 were added at the end of each section. As a consequence, the grouping of degradation methods was not maintained for the updated citations.

General methods exist for the decomposition or disposal of toxic organic chemicals. Such nonspecific procedures include catalytic oxidation, oxidation in a Parr bomb, the use of an oxygen plasma, incineration or combustion in furnaces specifically designed to minimize environmental contamination by flue gases, microbial degradation by activated sludges, and the disposal of bulk waste or adsorbed toxic materials by packaging, burial, etc. These methods are not practical for accidental laboratory spills, which must be decontaminated at the site by using (preferably) a procedure designed for the specific compound involved. In some cases, the disposal of small amounts of a toxic chemical may only require a simple hydrolysis; other compounds may require procedures for which more specialized laboratory equipment and knowledge for controlling reactions is necessary.

We acknowledge with pleasure the generous assistance and cooperation of the FCRC library staff, and the support of the National Cancer Institute under Contract No. NO1–CO–75380, with Litton Bionetics, Inc.

CONTENTS

Degradation
of
Chemical
Carcinogens

POLYCYCLIC AROMATIC HYDROCARBONS

POLYCYCLIC AROMATIC HYDROCARBONS*

Degradation Technique	Remarks	Reference
Oxidation	Evidence that certain diol epoxides are ultimate carcinogens suggests that oxidation products may be more hazardous than the parent compounds.	1
Oxidation	K-region oxidation products can be more mutagenic for mammalian cells than the parent compounds.	2
Oxidation	K-region oxidation products can be more efficient in transforming hamster embryo cells than the parent compounds.	3
Oxidation	A review, with 129 references, covering a large number of reagents and their mechanisms of action.	4
Oxidation	Ten polyclics were slowly oxidized by OsO_4 at ambient temperature to give the diols in good yields.	5
Oxidation	The formation of arene oxides, in high yields, occurred in 15 min to 24 hr at room temperature in the presence of NaOCl and tetrabutylammonium hydrogen sulfate at pH 8–9.	6
Oxidation	DBA and B(a)A were oxidized by DMSO; some other polyclics were not. Molecular O_2 was not needed to form quinones.	7
Oxidation	V_2O_5: polycyclic hydrocarbon (1:9) in 0.1N HCl caused degradation, which was greater in 0.1N HCl at elevated temperature. The carcinogenicity of MC was abolished. B(a)P and DMBA were included in the study.	8
Oxidation	Pyridinium iodide salts were obtained after oxidation with I_2 in the presence of pyridine at 30–35°C. B(a)A, DMBA, and MC yielded 54%, 58%, and 96%, respectively. Other polyclics were included in the study.	9

*See also specific compounds.

POLYCYCLIC AROMATIC HYDROCARBONS
(continued)

Degradation Technique	Remarks	Reference
Oxidation	The effects of pH, temperature, time, and concentration of chlorinating agent were determined for the degradation of B(a)A, B(a)P, and other polycyclic hydrocarbons in water. Toxicity of the products was not determined.	10
Ozonation	A detailed review of the chemistry of pyrene and its derivatives, including the degradation of pyrene by O_3.	11
Chemical	The synthesis and physicochemical properties of derivatives of five polycyclic aromatic hydrocarbons were reviewed. Carcinogenicity of the products was not discussed.	12
Photodecomposition	Minimizing photodegradation was briefly discussed in this review, concerned primarily with fluorescence analysis.	13
Photodecomposition	The effects of irradiation by sunlight, UV, and various fluorescent lamps were studied. Decomposition by UV was greater in the presence of O_2 than in the presence of N_2. DMBA, B(a)P, and B(a)A were included in the study.	14
Photodecomposition	A microbiological test for the carcinogenicity of polycyclic hydrocarbons was developed using *Tetrahymena pyriformis*. The UV degradation products from B(a)P still retained 50% of the original toxicity.	15
Reaction with maleic anhydride	Not a degradative procedure, but used in the preparation of derivatives for separating polycyclic hydrocarbons. B(a)A, MC, and DBA were included among reactive hydrocarbons.	16
Reaction with β-lactoglobulin	The *in vitro* transforming ability and toxicity of B(a)P for mouse kidney cells was inhibited by association with the protein.	17
Physicochemical Microbial	A review of recent work on the rates and methods of degradation of polycyclic hydrocarbons in wastewater.	18

POLYCYCLIC AROMATIC HYDROCARBONS
(continued)

Degradation Technique	Remarks	Reference
Microbial	Up to 55% of various polycyclics were oxidized by *Bacillus megaterium* in four days.	19
Microbial	A mutant strain of *Beijerinckia* oxidized B(a)P and B(a)A to the dihydrodiols.	20
Microbial	A strain of *Beijerinckia* catalyzed the incorporation of two atoms of O to form *cis*-dihydrodiols via a hypothetical dioxetane intermediate. B(a)P and B(a)A were included in the studies.	21
Microbial	A review, with 107 references, on the sources and biodegradation of carcinogenic hydrocarbons.	22

B(a)A: benz(a)anthracene   DMBA: 7,12-dimethylbenz(a)anthracene
B(a)P: benzo(a)pyrene   DMSO: dimethylsulfoxide
DBA: dibenzanthracene   MC: 3-methylcholanthrene

Polycyclic Aromatic Hydrocarbons

1. Lehr, R. E. and Jerina, D. M. Relationships of quantum mechanical calculations, relative mutagenicity of benzo(a)anthracene diol epoxides, and "bay region" concept of aromatic hydrocarbon carcinogenicity. *J. Toxicol. Environ. Health* 2:1259–1265, 1977.
2. Huberman, E., Aspiras, L., Heidelberger, C., Grover, P. L., and Sims, P. Mutagenicity to mammalian cells of epoxides and other derivatives of polycyclic hydrocarbons. *Proc. Natl. Acad. Sci.* 68:3195–3199, 1971.
3. Huberman, E., Kuroki, T., Marquardt, H., Selkirk, J. K., Heidelberger, C., Grover, P. L., and Sims, P. Transformation of hamster embryo cells by epoxides and other derivatives of polycyclic hydrocarbons. *Cancer Res.* 32:1391–1396, 1972.
4. Tipson, R. S. *Oxidation of Polycyclic, Aromatic Hydrocarbons. A Review of the Literature.* Natl. Bur. Stand. (U.S.) Monogr. 87, 52 pp., 1965.
5. Cook, J. W., and Schoental, R. Oxidation of carcinogenic hydrocarbons by osmium tetroxide. *J. Chem. Soc.*:170–173, 1948.
6. Krishnan, S., Kuhn, D. G., and Hamilton, G. A. Direct oxidation in high

yield of some polycyclic aromatic compounds to arene oxides using hypochlorite and phase transfer catalysts. *J. Am. Chem. Soc.* **99**:8121–8123,
1977.

7. Haga, J. J., Russell, B. R., and Chapel, J. F. Oxidation of several aromatic
   hydrocarbons using dimethyl sulfoxide exposed to the atmosphere. *Biochem. Biophys. Res. Commun.* **44**:521–525, 1971.

8. Gorski, T. The catalytic influence of V_2O_5 on the oxidation and on the
   disappearance of carcinogenic properties of some polycyclic hydrocarbons.
   Neoplasma **15**:267–271, 1968.

9. Cavalieri, E. and Roth, R. Reaction of methylbenzanthracenes and pyridine
   by one-electron oxidation. A model for metabolic activation and binding
   of carcinogenic aromatic hydrocarbons. *J. Org. Chem.* **41**:2679–2684,
   1976.

10. Harrison, R. M., Perry, R., and Wellings, R. A. Effect of water chlorination
    upon levels of some polynuclear aromatic hydrocarbons in water. *Environ.
    Sci. Technol.* **10**:1151–1156, 1976.

11. Vollmann, H., Becker, H., Corell, M., and Streeck, H. Pyrene and its de-
    rivatives. *Justus Liebigs Ann. Chem.* **531**:1–159, 1937.

12. McCaustland, D. J., Fischer, D. L., Kolwyck, K. C., Duncan, W. P., Wiley,
    J. C. Jr., Menon, C. S., Engel, J. F., Selkirk, J. K., and Roller, P. P. Poly-
    cyclic aromatic hydrocarbon derivatives: synthesis and physicochemical
    characterization. In: *Carcinogenesis–A Comprehensive Survey* **1**:349–411,
    Freudenthal, R. and Jones, P. W. (Eds.). Raven Press, New York, 1976.

13. Sawicki, E. Fluorescence analysis in air pollution research. *Talanta* **16**:
    1231–1266, 1969.

14. Kuratsune, M. and Hirohata, T. Decomposition of polycyclic aromatic
    hydrocarbons under laboratory illuminations. *Natl. Cancer Inst. Monogr.*
    9:117–125, 1962.

15. Gräf, W. and Haller, A. G. The phototoxic activity of carcinogenic poly-
    cyclic hydrocarbons and their degradation products in the biological test.
    Zentralbl. Bakteriol. Parasitenkd. Infektionskr. Hyg., Abt. 1: Orig., Reihe B
    164:250–261, 1977.

16. Jones, R. N., Gogek, C. J., and Sharpe, R. W. The reaction of maleic an-
    hydride with polynuclear aromatic hydrocarbons. *Can. J. Res.* **26**:719–727,
    1948.

17. Ono, J., Doi, K., Ogasa, K., and Nagasawa, T. Discrimination of carcino-
    genic activity and inactivation of transforming activity of hydrocarbons,
    by β-lactoglobulin. *Agric. Biol. Chem.* **39**:2149–2155, 1975.

18. Gubergrits, M. Mechanisms of natural and forced degradation of carcino-
    genic and toxic pollutants discharged into water bodies. *Vodn. Resur.*:185–
    188, 1975.

19. Fedoseeva, G. E., Khesina, A. Ya., Poglazova, M. N., Shabad, L. M., and
    Meisel, M. N. The oxidation of aromatic polycyclic hydrocarbons by micro-
    organisms. *Dokl. Akad. Nauk SSSR* **183**:208–211, 1968.

20. Gibson, D. T. Microbial degradation of polycyclic aromatic hydrocarbons. In: *Proceedings of the Third International Biodegradation Symposium:* 57–66, Sharpley, J. M. and Kaplan, A. M. (Eds.). Applied Science Publishers, London, 1976.
21. Gibson, D. T. Initial reactions in the bacterial degradation of aromatic hydrocarbons. *Zentralbl. Bakteriol. Parasitenkd. Infectionskr. Hyg., Abt. 1: Orig., Reihe B* 162:157–168, 1976.
22. ZoBell, C. E. Sources and biodegradation of carcinogenic hydrocarbons. In: *Proceedings of the Joint Conference on the Prevention and Control of Oil Spills:* 441–451. Am. Petrol. Inst., Washington, D.C., 1971.

BENZ(a)ANTHRACENE* (56-55-3)

Degradation Technique	Remarks	Reference
Reduction	Excess PtO_2 catalyst + H_2 (2 atm) at $25°C$ gave complete hydrogenation.	1
Reduction Oxidation	Quantitative hydrogenation occurred in glacial HOAc. Oxidation by $Na_2Cr_2O_7$ in HOAc gave the 7,12-quinone. Reacted as a diene in the Diels-Alder reaction.	2
Oxidation	A review, with 77 references, of the chemistry of B(a)A and its derivatives, including DMBA and MC. References were given for photo-oxidation and chemical oxidation by $Na_2Cr_2O_7$, $KMnO_4$, O_3, and OsO_4.	3
Oxidation	Treatment with Cl_2 for 6 hr in the presence of Tween 80 destroyed only about 31% of B(a)A. About 53% was destroyed in a mixture with other polycyclic hydrocarbons.	4
Oxidation	Oxidation products were identified after treatment with various reagents. Further derivatives were prepared and the properties of many related compounds were given.	5
Ozonation	The mechanism of O_3 attack and the effect of O_3 concentration on the products were studied. Included references to other oxidation reactions.	6
Photo-decomposition	B(a)A in 20% acetone in water required a threshold level of UV intensity for degradation. B(a)A was	7

*See also polycyclic aromatic hydrocarbons.

BENZ(a)ANTHRACENE (56-55-3)
(continued)

Degradation Technique	Remarks	Reference
	completely degraded to quinones, which were further decomposed. The studies included B(a)P and the effects of sunlight.	
Microbial	A mutant *Beijerinckia* species oxidized B(a)A and B(a)P to mixtures of vicinal dihydrodiols.	8
Microbial	B(a)A and other polycyclic hydrocarbons were oxidized to CO_2 during incubation for four days at $32°C$ with a marine bacterium. 47% of the theoretical yield of CO_2 was obtained with B(a)A and quantitative oxidation was predicted for longer incubations.	9

B(a)A: benz(a)anthracene   DMBA: 7,12-dimethylbenz(a)anthracene
B(a)P: benzo(a)pyrene   MC: 3-methylcholanthrene

Benz(a)anthracene

1. Jarman, M. Total reduction of benz(a)anthracene: the preparation of octa-decahydrobenz(a)anthracene. *Chem. Ind.* (London) 8:228, 1971.
2. *Int. Agency. Res. Cancer Monogr.* 3:45, Lyon, France, 1973.
3. Clar, E. *Polycyclic Hydrocarbons* 1:307-322. Academic Press, New York, 1964.
4. Scassellati Sforzolini, G., Saviano, A., and Merletti, L. Effect of chlorine on some polycyclic aromatic hydrocarbons. Destruction of carcinogenic compounds in water. *Boll. Soc. Ital. Biol. Sper.* 46:903-906, 1970.
5. Boyland, E. and Sims, P. Metabolism of polycyclic compounds. 24. The metabolism of benz(a)anthracene. *Biochem. J.* 91:493-506, 1964.
6. Moriconi, E. J., O'Connor, W. F., and Wallenberger, F. T. Ozonolysis of polycyclic aromatics. VI. Benz(a)anthracene and benz(a)anthracene-7, 12-dione. Correlation of quinone-hydroquinone oxidation-reduction potentials with the positions of predominant ozone attack. *J. Am. Chem. Soc.* 81:6466-6472, 1959.
7. McGinnes, P. R. and Snoeyink, V. L. *Determination of the fate of poly-nuclear aromatic hydrocarbons in natural water systems.* WRC Res. Rep. 80, University of Illinois Water Resources Center, Urbana, Illinois, 1974.

8. Gibson, D. T., Mahadevan, V., Jerina, D. M., Yagi, H., and Yeh, H. J. C. Oxidation of the carcinogens benzo(a)pyrene and benzo(a)anthracene to dihydrodiols by a bacterium. *Science* **189**:295–297, 1975.
9. Sisler, F. D. and ZoBell, C. E. Microbial utilization of carcinogenic hydrocarbons. *Science* **106**:521–522, 1947.

BENZO(a)PYRENE* (50-32-8)

Degradation Technique	Remarks	Reference
Photo-decomposition	UV irradiation in the presence of O_2 produced three quinones and smaller amounts of unidentified products.	1
Photo-decomposition	Long exposure of trace amounts to 254 nm UV was effective in a Petri dish. Most effective was UV on micelles of B(a)P in an aqueous detergent (complete in 4 hr).	2
Photo-decomposition	UV at 254 nm gave a product which produced abnormal mitoses in a chick embryo heart cell culture.	3
Photo-decomposition	Fluorescent light degraded B(a)P adsorbed on calcite and suspended in water. $T_{1/2}$ $(21°C, O_2)$ = 11 hr and decreased with increasing temperature.	4
Photo-decomposition	Several antioxidants enhanced the decomposition of B(a)P by long-wave UV light. B(a)P (1 $\mu g/ml$) was degraded by 20 hr of UV radiation to a greater extent in acetone (99.5%) than in water (54%) or hexane (40%).	5
Photo-decomposition	Low concentrations of B(a)P were degraded on TLC plates by UV; the rate depended on the degree of activation of the silica gel coating.	6
Photo-decomposition	A comparison was made of the degradation by fluorescent light of B(a)P in acetone solutions and while adsorbed on $CaCO_3$. The effects of pH, temperature, light intensity, O_2, ionic strength, and solvents were also studied. Products were not isolated.	7

*See also polycyclic aromatic hydrocarbons.

BENZO(a)PYRENE   (50–32–8)
(continued)

Degradation Technique	Remarks	Reference
Photo-decomposition	The products obtained after the irradiation of B(a)P with 365 nm light seemed not to be carcinogenic for mice.	8
Photo-decomposition	Of four solvents tested, dioxane gave the least stability under normal fluorescent lighting: complete loss of B(a)P in 22 hr in 25% (by volume in water) dioxane. Aqueous acetone solutions were the most stable.	9
Photo-decomposition	Studies in 20% aqueous acetone and in water indicated decomposition by UV to quinones, which were further degraded. Included data on B(a)A and the effects of sunlight.	10
Photo-decomposition	The loss of fluorescence produced by UV light was greater in acetone than in benzol solution.	11
Photo-decomposition	Degradation products (not identified) varied with the gas phase present during UV radiation in cyclohexane. X irradiation did not degrade B(a)P unless the solution in cyclohexane was finely dispersed in water.	12
Photo-decomposition	The presence of phenols inhibited the degradation of B(a)P in water reservoirs by natural photolysis.	13
Photo-decomposition	A kinetic study of B(e)P degradation in various solvents at $250^{\circ}C$ by UV radiation at 360 nm.	14
Photo-decomposition	The rate of photochemical oxidation of B(a)P was promoted by the presence of certain phenols.	15
Photo-decomposition	B(a)P was irradiated by UV or sunlight on thin silica gel layers or glass plates. Sunlight destroyed 65–95% in 5 hr on silica gel, but 100 times less on glass.	16
Photo-decomposition	Alkyl arylsulfonates increased the rate of photo-oxidation of B(a)P in water by increasing its solubility.	17
Photo-decomposition	B(a)P photolysis in acetone increased in the presence of 1,2-benzopyrene with an O_2 atmosphere.	18

BENZO(a)PYRENE (50-32-8)
(continued)

Degradation Technique	Remarks	Reference
Photo-decomposition	B(a)P was placed on thin silica gel layers and exposed to sunlight. A number of products formed and were compared with those obtained when the plates were stored in the dark.	19
Photo-decomposition	The effects of solvents, O_2, and temperature on the rate of B(a)P photodegradation were studied.	20
Photo-decomposition	B(a)P oxidation increased in the presence of DMBA (and *vice versa*). The effect was concentration and solvent dependent.	21
Photo-decomposition	The effects of B(a)P and phenols on the UV induced oxidation of each other were studied in the presence and absence of a sensitizer, eosin.	22
Photo-decomposition	3-Methylcholanthrene accelerated, and pyrene decreased the UV photolysis of B(a)P in benzene.	23
Photo-decomposition	A kinetic study of the degradation of B(a)P and its methyl derivatives by UV radiation of solutions in benzene or octane in the presence and absence of O_2 at $25°C$.	24
Photo-decomposition Thermal	Exposure to sunlight on silica gel gave at least 13 products (3 quinones) and 80% degradation of B(a)P. Similar tests were made with contaminated flour. The effect of baking was also studied, using dough containing B(a)P.	25
Photo-decomposition Oxidation Reduction	Various procedures gave at least four different free radicals which did not seem to react appreciably with antioxidants.	26
Photo-decomposition Ozonation Chlorination	Treatment with O_3 was more effective than treatment with Cl_2. UV irradiation was least effective in the removal of polycyclic hydrocarbons such as B(a)P and DMBA.	27
Photo-decomposition Ozonation	B(a)P was oxidized by UV light in the presence of O_2. The effectiveness varied with the solvent used. B(a)P was also oxidized by O_3. Many other polycyclic hydrocarbons were tested.	28

BENZO(a)PYRENE   (50-32-8)
(continued)

Degradation Technique	Remarks	Reference
Photo-decomposition Ozonation	Atmospheric conditions were simulated with O_3 and UV radiation. B(a)P, in very thin layers, had a $T_{1/2}$ of 5.3 hr in the presence of UV without O_3; 0.4 hr with 0.7 ppm O_3 in the absence of UV; and 0.2 hr with both O_3 and UV present.	29
Ozonation	A mixture of products formed, depending on the conditions of the reaction. Unreacted B(a)P was recovered in all cases.	30
Ozonation	B(a)P was treated with O_3 until its fluorescence was destroyed. The products were not toxic at 30 mg/rat.	31
Ozonation	Rapid decomposition of dilute aqueous solutions of B(a)P occurred with a mixture of air and O_3. Products were tested for carcinogenicity.	32
Ozonation	One mg of B(a)P was totally decomposed by 0.75 mg O_3. Six products were formed.	33
Ozonation	UV fluorescence, characteristic for B(a)P, was removed by 15–20 min treatment with O_3 of paraffins above their melting points (55–60°C), or of liquid paraffins at room temperature (20–30°C).	34
Ozonation Chlorination	Ozonation was much more effective than chlorination for the removal of B(a)P added to water samples.	35
Oxidation	Reacted with nucleophiles after oxidation by $Fe + H_2O_2$ or I_2 (57 references).	36
Oxidation	Oxidation by I_2 while adsorbed on silica gel gave products which reacted with nucleophiles (56 references).	37
Oxidation	B(a)P was destroyed by treating with hot dichromate cleaning solution. The work area was monitored with a UV lamp and kept free of fluorescence.	38
Oxidation	A bauxite catalyst was used for the rapid degradation of B(a)P in flue gases at 600°C.	39

BENZO(a) PYRENE (50-32-8)
(continued)

Degradation Technique	Remarks	Reference
Oxidation	Ten products were obtained by oxidation with H_2O_2 using a Pt catalyst. All of the B(a)P was oxidized in 24 hr at $65°C$, but the products were not identified.	40
Oxidation	A detailed study of the electrochemical oxidation of B(a)P, resulting mostly in a mixture of quinones, which were identified.	41
Oxidation	O_3 removed B(a)P and other carcinogens from water after mechanical purification, but it was suggested that impurities in industrial wastewater may be best destroyed in a cyclone furnace.	42
Oxidation	Waste gases were detoxified by combustion at $1500-1700°C$ or by catalytic oxidation at $450-500°C$.	43
Oxidation	A stack-type furnace was inadequate for destroying B(a)P in liquid industrial wastes. A vertical cyclone apparatus gave promising results.	44
Oxidation	B(a)P was completely removed from flue gases by catalytic oxidation at $550-600°C$.	45
Oxidation	Anodic oxidation of B(a)P in the presence of pyridine resulted in the formation of N-[6-benzo-(a)pyrenyl] pyridinium salt in high yield. Toxicity of this product was not discussed.	46
Oxidation	B(a)P in water was almost completely destroyed by Cl_2 treatment for 6 hr in the presence of Tween 80.	47
Oxidation	A kinetic study with metal oxide catalysts under various conditions.	48
Oxidation	Various reagents were tested for the oxygenation of B(a)P. Products were identified.	49
Oxidation	The diol-epoxide was found to be a tumor initiator in mice. References were made to other studies that showed that the diols of B(a)P and B(a)A were also potent initiators or mutagens.	50

BENZO(a) PYRENE (50-32-8)
(continued)

Degradation Technique	Remarks	Reference
Oxidation	A review of the chemistry of pyrene and its derivatives. Oxidation of B(a)P with chromic acid gave products which were identified.	51
Oxidation	A kinetic study of the oxidation of gaseous B(a)P over a V_2O_5-MoO_3 catalyst at 275–345°C.	52
Oxidation Microbial	Prevention of food contamination by industrial and automotive emitters was proposed by the use of anti-pollution methods (incineration, catalytic afterburners, filtration, etc.) and by the use of microorganisms for soil decontamination. A review with 31 references, no details.	53
Microbial	Soil bacteria adapted to B(a)P metabolism were able to degrade it (50–85% in four to five days). Other polycyclics also were degraded.	54
Microbial	Soil bacteria adapted to B(a)P metabolism destroyed B(a)P in culture media and in soil, but more degradation occurred in the presence of soil (82% in eight days at 28°C). Products were not identified.	55
Microbial	Degradation under "natural" conditions was greatest in soils that normally contained large amounts of B(a)P (up to 70% destroyed in three months).	56
Microbial	Considerable degradation of B(a)P (up to 60% in five days at 28°C) resulted when natural bacteria occurring in the contaminated water were supplemented with pure cultures of bacteria that oxidize polycyclic hydrocarbons. However, the wastewater was supplemented with meat-peptone broth during the incubations.	57
Microbial	Up to 85% degradation occurred in five days in soil cultures when bacteria isolated from contaminated soil were used.	58
Microbial	A mutant *Beijerinckia* species oxidized B(a)P and B(a)A to mixtures of vicinal dihydrodiols.	59

BENZO(a) PYRENE (50-32-8)
(continued)

Degradation Technique	Remarks	Reference
Microbial	B(a)P was effectively absorbed from wastewater by activated sludge.	60
Microbial	*Pseudomonas* species degraded B(a)P most rapidly in cultures in the stationary growth phase. Most of the data concerned studies with fluoranthene.	61
Microbial	B(a)P was usually completely degraded after 14–16 months in soil containing an anti-erosion agent.	62
Microbial Photo-decomposition	Laboratory model ecosystems were used for studying the bioaccumulation and degradation of B(a)P by various organisms. Only 8% was degraded by soil microbes in four weeks at $26.7°C$. Irradiation in methanol at 254 nm gave a $T_{1/2}$ of 2 hr.	63
Microbial Electrical discharge	The rate of degradation of B(a)P on activated sludge was about 18 times that induced by an electrical discharge; 75–99% of B(a)P was removed from wastewater by activated sludge in an aerated tank.	64
Electrical discharge	The kinetics of B(a)P degradation were studied during electrical discharge at the phase boundary of an aqueous solution.	65
Ionizing radiation	A kinetic study of the decomposition of B(a)P in nonaqueous solutions by ^{60}Co radiation. Products were identified.	66
Reaction with dimethyl acetylene-dicarboxylate	Apparently, several products rapidly formed during reaction at room temperature. The mixture was much less tumorigenic than B(a)P when injected (s.c.) into newborn rats.	67
Reduction	Total and partial hydrogenation were obtained with a PtO_2 catalyst at room temperature.	68
	After treatment by standard municipal water purification procedures, water usually did not contain more than 1–3 ng B(a)P/ℓ.	69

BENZO(a) PYRENE (50-32-8)
(continued)

Degradation Technique	Remarks	Reference
	A review (in Japanese) with 181 references on the activation and inactivation of B(a)P.	70

B(a)A: benz(a)anthracene
B(a)P: benzo(a)pyrene
B(e)P: benzo(e)pyrene
DMBA: 7,12-dimethylbenz(a)anthracene

Benzo(a)pyrene

1. Masuda, Y. and Kuratsune, M. Photochemical oxidation of benzo(a)pyrene. *Air Water Pollut. Int. J.* **10**:805–811, 1966.
2. Borneff, J. and Knerr, R. Carcinogenic substances in water and soil. II. Stability of 3,4-benzpyrene in light. *Arch. Hyg.* **143**:405–415, 1959.
3. Allsopp, C. B. Photo-oxides of carcinogenic hydrocarbons. *Nature* **145**:303, 1940.
4. Suess, M. J. Laboratory experimentation with 3,4-benzpyrene in aqueous systems and the environmental consequences. *Zentralbl. Bakteriol. Parasitenkd. Infectionskr. Hyg., Abt. 1: Orig., Reihe B* **155**:541–546, 1972.
5. Rondia, D. and Epstein, S. S. Effect of antioxidants on photodecomposition of benzo(a)pyrene. *Life Sci.* **7**:513–518, 1968.
6. Seifert, B. Stability of benzo(a)pyrene on silica gel plates for high-performance thin layer chromatography. *J. Chromatogr.* **131**:417–421, 1977.
7. Andelman, J. B. and Suess, M. J. The photodecomposition of 3,4-benzpyrene sorbed on calcium carbonate. In: *Organic Compounds in Aquatic Environments:* 439–468, Faust, S. J. and Hunter, J. V. (Eds.). Marcel Dekker, New York, 1971.
8. Gubergrits, M. Ya., Linnik, A. B., Paalme, L. P., and Shabad, L. M. The study of blastomogenicity of benzo(a)pyrene-photodegradation products. *Vopr. Onkol.* **20**:77–80, 1974.
9. Suess, M. J. Aqueous solutions of 3,4-benzpyrene. *Water Res.* **6**:981–985, 1972.
10. McGinnes, P. R. and Snoeyink, V. L. *Determination of the fate of polynuclear aromatic hydrocarbons in natural water systems.* WRC Res Rep 80, University of Illinois Water Resources Center, Urbana, Illinois, 1974.

11. Kriegel, H. and Herforth, L. Effect of long-wave UV light on the fluorescence of carcinogenic hydrocarbons in various solvents. II. The fluorescence stability of solutions at varying radiation intensities. *Z. Naturforsch., Teil B* 12:41–45, 1957.

12. Woenckhaus, J. W., Woenckhaus, C. W., and Koch, R. Studies on the effect of UV- and X-radiation on 3,4-benzpyrene. *Z. Naturforsch., Teil B* 17:295–299, 1962.

13. Gubergrits, M., Paalme, L., and Kirso, U. Degradation of benzo(a)pyrene and phenol by physicochemical agents during self-purification of reservoirs. *Vopr. Profil Zagryazeniya Vnesh Sredy, Chastnosti Vodoemov, Kantserogen Veshchestvami:* 49–53, 1972.

14. Paalme, L. and Gubergrits, M. Kinetics of photodecomposition of 1,2-benzopyrene. *Eesti NSV Tead Akad. Toim, Keem, Geol.* 21:48–52, 1972.

15. Karu, T., Kirso, U., and Gubergrits, M. Kinetics of the photoinduced cooxidation of benzo(a)pyrene and phenols. *Eesti NSV Tead Akad. Toim, Keem, Geol.* 22:217–223, 1973.

16. Mailath, F. P., Medve, F., and Morik, J. Photolysis of 3,4-benzpyrene by ultraviolet radiation and sunlight. *Egeszsegtudomany* 18:333–341, 1974.

17. Paalme, L., Priiman, R., Glushko, M. I., and Gubergrits, M. Simultaneous photoinduced oxidation of 3,4-benzpyrene and alkyl arylsulfonates. *Vodn. Resur.:* 174–178, 1975.

18. Paalme, L. and Gubergrits, M. Kinetics of cooxidation of 1,2- and 3,4-benzopyrenes activated by UV radiation. In: *Teor Prakt Zhidkofazn Okisleniya:* 12–122, Emanuel, N. M. (Ed.). "Nauka," Moscow, USSR, 1974.

19. Mailath, F. P. and Morik, J. Thin-layer chromatography of photooxidation of 3,4-benzopyrene. *Egeszsegtudomany* 19:277–284, 1975.

20. Paalme, L. and Gubergrits, M. Factors affecting the photodegradation of benzo(a)pyrene. *Vopr. Profil Zagryaz Okruzhayushchei Chel Sredy Kantserogennymi Veshchestvami:* 19–21, 1972.

21. Paalme, L., Lopp, A., and Gubergrits, M. Kinetics of cooxidative photodegradation of benzo(a)pyrene and 7,12-dimethylbenz(a)anthracene. *Eesti NSV Tead Akad. Toim, Keem, Geol.* 25:247–249, 1976.

22. Kirso, U. and Gubergrits, M. Photo-induced cooxidation kinetics of 3,4-benzopyrene, phenol, and 5-methylresorcinol. *Eesti NSV Tead Akad. Toim, Keem, Geol.* 20:134–140, 1971.

23. Paalme, L. and Gubergrits, M. Kinetics of the separate and combined photodegradation of benzo(a)pyrene, pyrene, and 3-methylcholanthrene. *Eesti NSV Tead Akad. Toim, Keem, Geol.* 25:271–275, 1976.

24. Paalme, L., Perin-Roussel, O., Gubergrits, M., and Jacquignon, P. Relation between structure and reactivity of benzo(a)pyrene and some of its methyl derivatives. *J. Chim. Phys. Phys.-Chim. Biol.* 74:496–498, 1977.

25. Rohrlich, M. and Suckow, P. Oxidative modification of 3,4-benzpyrene on cereals and in pastry. *Chem. Mikrobiol. Technol. Lebensm.* 2:137–143, 1973.

26. Menger, E. M., Spokane, R. B., and Sullivan, P. D. Free radicals derived from benzo(a)pyrene. *Biochem. Biophys. Res. Commun.* 71:610–616, 1976.

27. Il'nitskii, A. P., Ershova, K. P., Khesina, A. Ya., Rozhkova, L. G., Klubkov, V. G., and Korolev, A. A. Stability of carcinogenic substances in water and the efficacy of methods of decontamination. *Gig. Sanit.* 36(4):8–12, 1971.

28. Boyland, E. Studies in tissue metabolism. II. The inhibition of lactic dehydrogenase by derivatives of carcinogenic compounds. *Biochem. J.* 27: 791–801, 1933.

29. Lane, D. A. and Katz, M. The photomodification of benzo(a)pyrene, benzo(b)fluoranthene, and benzo(k)fluoranthene under simulated atmospheric conditions. In: *Fate of Pollutants in the Air and Water Environments, Part 2:* 137–154, Suffet, I. H. (Ed.). John Wiley & Sons, New York, 1977.

30. Moriconi, E. J., Rakoczy, B., and O'Connor, W. F. Ozonolysis of polycyclic aromatics. VIII. Benzo(a)pyrene. *J. Am. Chem. Soc.* 83:4618–4623, 1961.

31. Szollosi, E., Morik, J., Szitar, E., Tumpek, J., Jakucs, E., and Tatar-Kiss, Z. Studies on the chronic toxicity of ozone degraded 3,4-benzpyrene products. *Egeszsegtudomany* 20:187–193, 1976.

32. Korolev, A. A. and Il'nitskii, A. P. Effectiveness of ozonization of water containing petroleum products and benzo(a)pyrene. *Vopr. Profil Zagryazneniya Vnesh Sredy, Chastnosti Vodoemov, Kantserogen Veshchestv:* 40–43, 1972.

33. Mailath, F. P., Medve, F., Morik, J., and Nagy, Z. Decomposition of 3,4-benzpyrene by ozone. *Egeszsegtudomany* 19:65–71, 1975.

34. Goryaev, M. I., Ignatova, L. A., Artamonov, A. F., and Kocheva, Z. V. Removal of carcinogenic substances from paraffinic hydrocarbons. *Izv. Akad. Nauk Kaz. SSR, Ser. Khim.* 26(5):80–81, 1976.

35. Gabovich, R. D., Kurennoi, I. L., and Fedorenko, Z. P. Effect of ozone and chlorine on 3,4-benzopyrene during the disinfection of water. *Gig. Naselennykh Mest.* 8:88–91, 1969.

36. Cavalieri, E. and Auerbach, R. Reactions between activated benzo(a)-pyrene and nucleophilic compounds, with possible implications on the mechanism of tumor initiation. *J. Natl. Cancer Inst.* 53:393–397, 1974.

37. Wilk, M. and Girke, W. Reactions between benzo(a)pyrene and nucleobases by one-electron oxidation. *J. Natl. Cancer Inst.* 49:1585–1597, 1972.

38. Mulik, J., Cooke, M., Guyer, M. F., Seminiuk, G. M., and Sawicki, E. A gas liquid chromatographic fluorescent procedure for the analysis of benzo(a)pyrene in 24 hour atmospheric particulate samples. *Anal. Lett.* 8:511–524, 1975.

39. Mezhuev, M. I., Gorshkov, V. S., and Khesina, A. Ya. Use of a catalytic burning method to remove 3,4-benzopyrene from industrial gases. *Gig. Sanit.* 38(6):102–104, 1973.

40. Biondi, A. *In vitro* oxidation of 3,4-benzopyrene: chromatographic separation of the oxidation products. *Rass. Med. Sper.* 21:82–89, 1974.
41. Jeftic, L. and Adams, R. N. Electrochemical oxidation pathways of benzo(a)pyrene. *J. Am. Chem. Soc.* 92:1332–1337, 1970.
42. Shkodin, P. E., Gracheva, M. P., Tikhomirov, Yu. P., and Baikovskii, V. V. Comparative evaluation of effectiveness of some methods for wastewater decarcinogenation. *Gig. Sanit.* 40(1):13–15, 1975.
43. Abaseev, V. K. Thermal and catalytic detoxification of waste gases containing 3,4-benzopyrene. *Khim. Prom.* 49:25–26, 1973.
44. Baikovskii, V. V. Hygienic characteristics of a method of fire detoxification for liquid industrial wastes. *Gig. Sanit.* 39(12):88–89, 1974.
45. Foksha, G. A. Detoxification of bitumen industry flue gases by catalytic oxidation. *Prom. Sanit. Ochistka Gazov* (2):12, 1976.
46. Blackburn, G. M. and Will, J. P. Bonding of benzo(a)pyrene to nitrogen heterocycles by anodic oxidation. *J. Chem. Soc. Chem. Commun.* (2):67–68, 1974.
47. Scassellati Sforzolini, G., Saviano, A., and Merletti, L. Effect of chlorine on some polycyclic aromatic hydrocarbons. Destruction of carcinogenic compounds in water. *Boll. Soc. Ital. Biol. Sper.* 46:903–906, 1970.
48. Young, G. W. Kinetic modelling for the catalytic oxidation of benzo(a)pyrene. *Diss. Abstr. Int. B* 37:4581–4582, 1977.
49. Ioki, Y. and Nagata, C. A fluorimetric and electron spin resonance study of oxygenation of benzo(a)pyrene; an interpretation of the enzymic oxygenation. *J. Chem. Soc., Perkin Trans.* 2:1172–1175, 1977.
50. Slaga, T. J., Viaje, A., Bracken, W. M., Berry, D. L., Fischer, S. M., Miller, D. R., and Leclerc, S. M. Skin-tumor-initiating ability of benzo(a)pyrene-7,8-diol-9,10-epoxide (anti) when applied topically in tetrahydrofuran. *Cancer Lett.* 3:23–30, 1977.
51. Vollman, H., Becker, H., Corell, M., and Streeck, H. Pyrene and its derivatives. *Ann. Chem.* 531:1–159, 1937.
52. Young, G. W., and Greene, H. L. Kinetic modeling for the catalytic oxidation of benzo(a)pyrene. *J. Catal.* 50:258–267, 1977.
53. Fritz, W. and Engst, R. On environmental contamination of foods with carcinogenic hydrocarbons. *Z. Gesamte Hyg. Ihre Grenzgeb.* 17:271–275, 1971.
54. Shabad, L. M., Cohan, Y. L., Ilnitsky, A. P., Khesina, A. Ya., Shcherbak, N. P., and Smirnov, G. A. The carcinogenic hydrocarbon benzo(a)pyrene in the soil. *J. Natl. Cancer Inst.* 47:1179–1191, 1971.
55. Poglazova, M. N., Fedoseeva, G. E., Khesina, A. Ya., Meisel, M. N., and Shabad, L. M. Destruction of benzo(a)pyrene by soil bacteria. *Life Sci.* 6:1053–1062, 1967.
56. Khesina, A. Ya., Shcherbak, N. P., Shabad, L. M., and Vostrov, I. S. Benzpyrene breakdown by the soil microflora. *Byull. Eksp. Biol. Med.* 68(10):70–73, 1969.

57. Poglazova, M. N., Khesina, A. Ya., Fedoseeva, G. E., Meisel, M. N., and Shabad, L. M. The microbial degradation of benz(a)pyrene in wastewaters. *Dokl. Akad. Nauk SSSR* 204:222–225, 1972.
58. Poglazova, M. N., Fedoseeva, G. E., Khesina, A. Ya., Meisel, M. N., and Shabad, L. M. Metabolism of benz(a)pyrene by various soil microflora and isolated microorganisms. *Dokl. Akad. Nauk SSSR* 198:1211–1213, 1971.
59. Gibson, D. T., Mahadevan, V., Jerina, D. M., Yagi, H., and Yeh, H. J. C. Oxidation of the carcinogens benzo(a)pyrene and benzo(a)anthracene to dihydrodiols by a bacterium. *Science* 189:295–297, 1975.
60. Samoilovich, L. M., Trubnikov, V. Z., Matsieva, E. M., and Nemzer, V. G. Effectiveness of decontaminating wastewaters containing 3,4-benzpyrene on biological treatment plants. *Gig. Sanit.* 40(10):98–99, 1975.
61. Barnsley, E. A. The bacterial degradation of fluoranthene and benzo(a)-pyrene. *Can. J. Microbiol.* 21:1004–1008, 1975.
62. Kogan, Yu. L. Dynamics of benzo(a)pyrene breakdown in various types of soils. *Gig. Sanit.* 39(7):110–113, 1974.
63. Lu, P.-Y., Metcalf, R. L., Plummer, N., and Mandel, D. The environmental fate of three carcinogens: benzo(a)pyrene, benzidine, and vinyl chloride evaluated in laboratory model ecosystems. *Arch. Environ. Contam. Toxicol.* 6:129–142, 1977.
64. Gubergrits, M., Hannus, M., Brodskaya, B. Kh., Kirso, U., and Paalme, L. Use of processes for activated oxidative degradation of benzo(a)pyrene in water. In: *Mater Vses Nauchn Simp Sovrem Probl Samoochisncheniya Regul Kach Vody, 5th* 6:109, 1975.
65. Brodskaya, B. Kh., Paalme, L., and Gubergrits, M. Evaluation of the effect of electrical discharge by the use of model reactions in liquid phase. I. Degradation of 3,4-benzopyrene in an aqueous solution under discharge at the phase boundary. *Eesti NSV Tead Akad. Toim, Keem, Geol.* 24:301–303, 1975.
66. Uibopuu, H., Gubergrits, M. Ya., and Rajavaa, E. Oxidative liquid-phase γ-radiolysis of 3,4-benzopyrene. *Latv. PSR Zinat Akad. Vestis* (3):116–118, 1973.
67. Iwanami, Y. and Odashima, S. Inactivation of benzo(a)pyrene. *Naturwissenschaften* 61:509, 1974.
68. Lijinsky, W. and Zechmeister, L. On the catalytic hydrogenation of 3,4-benzpyrene. *J. Am. Chem. Soc.* 75:5495–5497, 1953.
69. Il'nitskii, A. P., Sherenesheva, N. I., and Kutakov, K. V. Efficiency of decontamination of water containing benzopyrene in water treatment installations. *Gig. Sanit.* 37(11):24–26, 1972.
70. Nemoto, N. Activation and inactivation mechanisms of benzo(a)pyrene. *Tampakushitsu Kakusan Koso* 21:957–971, 1976.

7-BROMOMETHYLBENZ(a)ANTHRACENE (24961-39-5)

Degradation Technique	Remarks	Reference
Reaction with 4-(p-nitro-benzyl)-pyridine	$T_{1/2}$ was 2.2 min at 49.5°C, but varied with the concentration of the reagent.	1
Reaction with nucleophiles	The reactions with nucleic acids, polynucleo-tides, and nucleosides were studied in aqueous and in dimethylacetamide solutions.	2

7-Bromomethylbenz(a)anthracene

1. Dipple, A. and Slade, T. A. Structure and activity in chemical carcinogenesis: reactivity and carcinogenicity of 7-bromomethylbenz(a)anthracene and 7-bromomethyl-12-methylbenz(a)anthracene. *Eur. J. Cancer* **6**:417–423, 1970.
2. Dipple, A., Brookes, P., Mackintosh, D. S., and Rayman, M. P. Reaction of 7-bromomethylbenz(a)anthracene with nucleic acids, polynucleotides and nucleosides. *Biochemistry* **10**:4323–4330, 1971.

7,12-DIMETHYLBENZ(a)ANTHRACENE (57-97-6)

Degradation Technique	Remarks	Reference
Photo-decomposition	Variable degradation occurred in 12–124 hr with varied type and level of light. Several products were obtained; one was carcinogenic. No details.	1
Photo-decomposition	The loss of fluorescence was proportional to the UV dosage and was greater in acetone than in benzol. Included data with benzo(a)pyrene.	2
Photo-decomposition	The main product of UV radiation was the 7,12-epoxide. Rate of oxidation was affected by the solvent, wavelength, and intensity.	3
Photo-decomposition	DMBA photo-oxidation increased in the presence of benzo(a)pyrene (and *vice versa*). The effect was concentration and solvent dependent.	4

7,12-DIMETHYLBENZ(a)ANTHRACENE (57-97-6)
(continued)

Degradation Technique	Remarks	Reference
Oxidation	Oxidation with lead tetraacetate formed acetoxy-methyl derivatives. No details.	5
Oxidation	The ascorbic acid-Fe^{+2} -O_2 model system resulted in the formation of several products, but only a few were identified. The reaction was incomplete in 24 hr at room temperature.	6
Oxidation Ozonation	Oxidation with $Na_2 Cr_2 O_7$ gave the quinone in good yield. Ozonation resulted in a mixture which was oxidized with $H_2 O_2$ or $Ag_2 O$. The products were identified.	7

DMBA: 7,12-dimethylbenz(a)anthracene

7,12-Dimethylbenz(a)anthracene

1. Davies, R. E. Destruction of 7,12-dimethylbenz(a)anthracene (DMBA) by ambient light. *Proc. Am. Assoc. Cancer Res.* 12:31, 1971.
2. Kriegel, H. and Herforth, L. The effect of long wave UV light on the fluorescence of carcinogenic hydrocarbons in various solvents. II. The fluorescence stability of solutions at various radiation intensities. *Z. Naturforsch., Teil B* 12:41–45, 1957.
3. Lopp, A., Paalme, L., and Gubergrits, M. Kinetics of photoinitiated oxidation of 7,12-dimethylbenz(a)anthracene in various solvents. *Eesti NSV Tead Akad. Toim, Keem, Geol.* 25:22–27, 1976.
4. Paalme, L., Lopp, A., and Gubergrits, M. Kinetics of cooxidative photodegradation of benzo(a)pyrene and 7,12-dimethylbenz(a)anthracene. *Eesti NSV Tead Akad. Toim, Keem, Geol.* 25:247–249, 1976.
5. Pataki, J. and Balick, R. Oxidation of 7,8,12-trimethylbenz(a)anthracene with lead tetraacetate. *Tetrahedron Lett.* 38:3447–3449, 1974.
6. Boyland, E. and Sims, P. Metabolism of polycyclic compounds: the metabolism of 7,12-dimethylbenz(a)anthracene by rat-liver homogenates. *Biochem. J.* 95:780–787, 1965.
7. Moriconi, E. J. and Taranko, L. B. Ozonolysis of polycyclic aromatics. X. 7,12-dimethylbenz(a)anthracene. *J. Org. Chem.* 28:1831–1834, 1963.

3-METHYLCHOLANTHRENE (56-49-5)

Degradation Technique	Remarks	Reference
Photo-decomposition	Oxidation in the light of a 60 W bulb for 48 hr at 25°C was catalyzed by dimethylsulfoxide. Five products were identified (plus some un-changed MC).	1
Oxidation	Oxidation was catalyzed by V_2O_5 at 37°C in 0.1 N HCl in acetone solution to produce quinones.	2
Oxidation	Various products were obtained when MC was treated with O_3, H_2O_2, or $H_2Cr_2O_7$. References were given for other chemical reactions of MC.	3
Oxidation	Products were identified after oxidation by singlet oxygen generated chemically or photo-chemically.	4

MC: 3-Methylcholanthrene

3-Methylcholanthrene

1. Dao, T. L., King, C., and Tominaga, T. Isolation, identification and biological study of compounds derived from 3-methylcholanthrene by irradiation in dimethyl sulfoxide. *Cancer Res.* 31:1492–1495, 1971.
2. Gorski, T. and Krzywanska, E. Electron spin resonance study of the free radicals of 3-methylcholanthrene oxi-derivatives. *Pol. Med. Sci. Hist. Bull.* 12:136–138, 1969.
3. Moriconi, E. J. and Taranko, L. B. Ozonolysis of polycyclic aromatics. XI. 3-Methylcholanthrene. *J. Org. Chem.* 28:2526–2529, 1963.
4. Frazer, J. M. Chemiluminescent display of electronic excitation state generation from the oxidation of 3-methylcholanthrene by singlet molecular oxygen. *Diss. Abstr. Int. B* 30:4559–4560, 1970.

NITROSAMINES AND NITROSAMIDES

NITROSAMINES AND NITROSAMIDES*

Degradation Technique	Remarks	Reference
	A note warning that nitrosamides can explode, decompose slowly, or polymerize.	1
Reduction	Fifteen ppm solutions of NDEA, NDMA, NPIP, and NPYR were efficiently reduced by Al + NaOH. See NDMA #1 for warning.	2
Reduction	Nitrosamines were reduced to hydrazines by refluxing with LiAlH$_4$ in tetrahydrofuran. The hydrazines were reacted with 9-anthraldehyde to form hydrazones. Basis for analysis.	3
Reduction	Electrochemical reduction produced amines which were derivatized for GLC analysis of nitrosamines in foods.	4
Reduction	Preparative electrochemical reduction of nitrosamines at pH 1 or pH 5 gave the corresponding asymmetric hydrazines. At alkaline pH, secondary amines and N$_2$O were formed.	5
Reduction	Conditions for the electrolysis of alkyl nitrosamines were controlled to yield mostly unsymmetric alkylhydrazines or alkylamines.	6
Photo-decomposition	Fifteen min UV irradiation under specified conditions gave 95–100% degradation of nitrosamines, but only 31–71% for nitrosamides. Basis for colorimetric procedure (HNO$_2$ released).	7
Photo-decomposition	The release of nitrite from nitrosamines by UV irradiation at alkaline pH was used as a method for analysis.	8
Photo-decomposition	NDMA and NDEA were included in a method for analyzing N-nitroso compounds by photolysis to release nitrite quantitatively at pH 7.	9

*See also specific compounds.

NITROSAMINES AND NITROSAMIDES
(continued)

Degradation Technique	Remarks	Reference
Photo-decomposition	Possible mechanisms were considered for the intermediate steps in the degradation of nitrosamines.	10
Photo-decomposition	$T_{1/2}$ determined for NDMA, NDBA, and NPIP during UV irradiation at different pH's and in different solvents.	11
Photo-decomposition	UV (366 nm) irradiation of nitrosamines in KOH produced nitrite. Basis for analysis.	12
Photo-decomposition	UV irradiation in an acidic solution resulted in the photoaddition of nitrosamines to cyclic olefins. NPIP and NDMA were studied.	13
Photo-decomposition	UV irradiation of nitrosamines on activated silica gel TLC plates produced primary amines, which were detected by fluorescamine.	14
Photo-decomposition	Several nitrosamines were degraded by sunlight: $T_{1/2}$ for NDEA was 9.5 hr; for DNPZ, it was 3 hr. An LD50 or LD100 dose of NDEA had no toxic effect on rats after photolysis of the solution.	15
Photo-decomposition	The photolysis of nitrosamines was studied under varied conditions. Products were identified.	16
Photo-decomposition	Nitrosamines were destroyed by 366 nm UV irradiation; efficiency varied with the solvent used. Part of a GLC analytical method.	17
Photo-decomposition	Nitrosamines in air samples were completely adsorbed by a microporous membrane. They were then eluted, decomposed by UV irradiation, and the NO_2 measured by diazotization.	18
Hydrolysis	Seventeen nitrosamines tested gave 99.5% denitrosation by HBr in glacial HOAc. Nitrosamides were more stable. Part of a procedure for colorimetric analysis: 15 min at 20°C or 3 min at 50°C gave complete degradation of NDMA. See NDMA #1 for warning.	19

NITROSAMINES AND NITROSAMIDES
(continued)

Degradation Technique	Remarks	Reference
Hydrolysis	HBr in glacial HOAc released HNO_2 in high yields even from nonvolatile nitrosamines and nitrosamides.	20
Hydrolysis	Rate constants were determined for the hydrolyses of alkyl nitrosoureas at pH 6–7.8 and at 30–40°C. $T_{1/2}$ was 32 min for MNU at pH 6.8, 35°C.	21
Hydrolysis	Nitrosamides were degraded when heated for 45 min in dilute HCl. The HNO_2 released was determined colorimetrically. Nitrosamines did not react under the conditions used.	22
Hydrolysis	$T_{1/2}$ of MNU and ENU determined at pH 5–7.9 at 37°C (some data at 15°C). NDMA and NDEA did not degrade in 4 hr.	23
Hydrolysis	Complete hydrolysis of unbuffered solutions of nitrosamides at 25°C in the dark occurred in 72–504 hr as estimated by seedling height reduction.	24
Hydrolysis	$T_{1/2}$ for NDMA, MNU, MNUT, and NMTS at pH 7, 20°C and 37°C, cited from published data. $T_{1/2}$ for MNU was 32 min at 37°C and 3.5 hr at 20°C in saline/citrate solution (final pH 6.6).	25
Hydrolysis	Dialkylnitrosamines were cleaved in various ways by "superacid solutions" at 80–140°C.	26
Hydrolysis	Cu^{+2} markedly stimulated the hydrolysis of ENU, MNU, and especially MNNG at pH 6, 37°C. Cu^{+2} inhibited the hydrolysis of MNUT.	27
Hydrolysis	Various nitrosamides were shown to release HNO_2 at pH 2.2–2.3.	28
Hydrolysis	Rate constants were determined at alkaline pH for MNUT, ENUT, and several β-alkyl nitrosaminoketones.	29

NITROSAMINES AND NITROSAMIDES
(continued)

Degradation Technique	Remarks	Reference
Hydrolysis	The kinetics of acid hydrolysis of nitroso derivatives of secondary amines were studied. HCl was more effective than other acids tested.	30
Oxidation	$H_2O_2 + CF_3COOH$ oxidized nitrosamines to nitramines in good yields.	31
Oxidation	Secondary nitrosamines were quantitatively oxidized to nitramines by CF_3CO_3H in CH_2Cl_2. This was preferred to the use of CF_3COOH and H_2O_2.	32
Oxidation	CF_3CO_3H was used to oxidize volatile nitrosamines to nitramines as a basis for GLC analysis of foodstuff contamination.	33
Oxidation	The efficiency of conversion of nitrosamines to nitramines by CF_3CO_3H was determined.	34
Oxidation	Nitrosamines were converted to nitramines by oxidation with CF_3CO_3H.	35
Oxidation	Refluxing nitrosamines with 2-butanone peroxide gave the corresponding nitramines.	36
Oxidation Photo-decomposition	Fenton's reagent ($Fe^{+2} + H_2O_2$) and alkaline peroxydisulfate had no effect on the nitrosamines tested. Oxidation by Udenfriend's hydroxylase model (ascorbic acid + Fe^{+2} + EDTA + O_2) produced derivatives which retained the nitrosamine group. UV irradiation in water or aqueous H_2O_2 caused hydrolysis with the formation of secondary amines and NO^{-2} or NO_3^-. Rate constants and $T_{1/2}$ were determined.	37
Photo-decomposition Hydrolysis	Acid was needed for good photolysis. NDBA and NPIP were included in the studies. Products were determined. Hydrolysis did not occur beyond 10–12% in 24 hr of refluxing in 0.5N HCl.	38
Photo-decomposition Hydrolysis	$T_{1/2}$ determined for MNNG, MNU, MNUT, and NMTS when irradiated with fluorescent light at pH 5, $26°C$. $T_{1/2}$ determined for the degradation of the same compounds at $37°C$ and pH 2–9.	39

NITROSAMINES AND NITROSAMIDES
(continued)

Degradation Technique	Remarks	Reference
Hydrolysis Reduction Oxidation Photo-decomposition	Included in a review of nitrosamines in foodstuffs.	40
Hydrolysis Reduction Oxidation Photo-decomposition	A review, with 272 references, giving chemical properties and degradative reactions for aliphatic nitrosamines.	41
Hydrolysis Reduction Oxidation Photo-decomposition	A review with nine references. No details	42
Hydrolysis Reduction Oxidation Photo-decomposition	A definitive study relating chemical structure and carcinogenicity of 65 N-nitroso compounds. Gave properties, including water-stability, of many of the compounds, and rates of hydrolysis of nitrosamides at various pH's. 149 references.	43
Hydrolysis Reaction with nucleophiles	$T_{1/2}$ for MNU or ENU was 10 min at 25°C and pH 8. Reactions with $S_2O_3{}^{-2}$, thiourea, I^-, SCN^-, and Cl^- were studied.	44
Physical Chemical	A review including the chemistry and metabolism of N-nitroso compounds.	45
Thermal	The N-NO bond was broken in a noncatalytic pyrolyzer at 300–500°C. Part of a chromatographic detection system.	46
Thermal	N-Alkyl-N-nitrosamides were converted to N_2 and the corresponding esters by heating for 10–15 hr in nonpolar solvents at relatively low temperatures.	47

NITROSAMINES AND NITROSAMIDES
(continued)

Degradation Technique	Remarks	Reference
Microbial	NDMA, NDEA, and NDPA were all resistant to microbial degradation. But see #49 and #50.	48
Microbial	NDMA, NDEA, and NDPA were resistant to bacterial degradation. They were degraded slowly in soil and sewage, but not in lake water in 3.5 months.	49
Microbial	The degradations of NDMA, NPYR, and NDPHA were studied, using bacteria isolated from rat intestines. Secondary amines and nitrite were formed.	50
Ozonation	Nitrosamines were resistant to conventional municipal water treatments, but were degraded by ozonation at alkaline pH.	51
Photo-decomposition	Two prototype apparatuses were described for the degradation of nitrosamines using NDMA as a model compound. One instrument, using fluorescent lamps, destroyed about 0.01 mole of NDMA in 24 hr; the other, using UV radiation, degraded about 0.15 mole. Degradation was most efficient at low pH values. The addition of NO_2^--scavengers was necessary to prevent the resynthesis of nitrosamines after irradiation, and especially before releasing the products into the sewage system. Hydrazoic acid was the best scavenging agent tested; urea and guanidine were less efficient.	52
Hydrolysis	HNO_2 or secondary amines released by acid were used for the colorimetric detection of micro amounts of N-nitrosamines and nitrosamides. This might be applied as a method of monitoring surface contamination.	53
Hydrolysis	Denitrosation occurred in acid in the presence of a halide or SCN^- and a nitrite scavenger. I^- was about 15,000 times more reactive than Cl^-.	54

NITROSAMINES AND NITROSAMIDES
(continued)

Degradation Technique	Remarks	Reference
Hydrolysis Reaction with 4-(p-nitrobenzyl)-pyridine	The rates of decomposition of several nitrosourea derivatives were determined in cacodylate buffer, pH 7.0, at 37°C. $T_{1/2}$ for MNU was 27.6 min; for ENU, 34.1 min. The alkylating activity of mono-N-nitrosoureas at pH 6.0 and 37°C decreased with increasing length of the alkyl chain.	55
Reduction	Several nitrosamines were rapidly converted to NO and the corresponding secondary bases by treatment with a cold solution of CuCl in HCl.	56

DNPZ:	N-dinitrosopiperazine		NDEA:	N-nitrosodiethylamine
ENU:	N-nitrosoethylurea		NDMA:	N-nitrosodimethylamine
ENUT:	N-nitrosoethylurethane		NDPA:	N-nitrosodipropylamine
MNNG:	N-methyl-N'-nitro-N-nitrosoguanidine		NDPHA:	N-nitrosodiphenylamine
			NMTS:	N-nitrosomethyl-p-tolylsulfonamide
MNU:	N-nitrosomethylurea			
MNUT:	N-nitrosomethylurethane		NPIP:	N-nitrosopiperidine
NDBA:	N-nitrosodibutylamine		NPYR:	N-nitrosopyrrolidine

Nitrosamines and Nitrosamides

1. Lijinsky, W. Instability of N-nitrosamides. *Science* 183:368, 1974.
2. Gangolli, S. D., Shilling, W. H., and Lloyd, A. G. A method for the destruction of nitrosamines in solution. *Food Cosmet. Toxicol.* 12:168, 1974.
3. Yank, K. W. and Brown, E. V. A sensitive analysis for nitrosamines. *Anal. Lett.* 5:293–304, 1972.
4. Alliston, T. G., Cox, G. B., and Kirk, R. S. The determination of steam-volatile N-nitrosamines in foodstuffs by formation of electron-capturing derivatives from electrochemically derived amines. *Analyst (London)* 97:915–920, 1972.
5. Lund, H. Electroorganic preparations. III. Polarography and reduction of N-nitrosamines. *Acta Chem. Scand.* 11:990–996, 1957.
6. Whitnack, C. G., Weaver, R. D., and Kruse, H. W. *Polarographic Behavior and Large-Scale Electrolysis of Some Alkylnitrosamines.* NOTS Technical

Publication **3253**, U.S. Naval Ordnance Test Station, China Lake, California, 1963.

7. Daiber, D. and Preussmann, R. Quantitative colorimetric determination of organic N-nitroso compounds by photochemical cleavage of the nitrosamine bond. *Z. Anal. Chem.* **206**:344–352, 1964.
8. Walters, C. L., Johnson, E. M., and Ray, N. Separation and detection of volatile and non-volatile N-nitrosamines. *Analyst (London)* **95**:485–489, 1970.
9. Fan, T.-Y. and Tannenbaum, S. R. Automatic colorimetric determination of N-nitroso compounds. *J. Agric., Food Chem.* **19**:1267–1269, 1971.
10. Burgess, E. M. and Lavanish, J. M. Photochemical decomposition of N-nitrosamines. *Tetrahedron Lett.* 1221–1226, 1964.
11. Burns, D. T. and Alliston, G. V. Some studies on the photolytic decomposition stage in the estimation of N-nitrosamines. *J. Food Technol.* **6**:433–438, 1971.
12. Sander, J. A method for the detection of nitrosamines. *Hoppe-Seyler's Z. Physiol. Chem.* **348**:852–854, 1967.
13. Chow, Y. L., Chen, S. C., Pillay, K. S., and Perry, R. A. Photoreactions of nitroso compounds in solution. XXI. Stereochemical course of photoaddition of nitrosamines to some cyclic olefins and conformational isomers generated by $A^{1,3}$-interaction. *Can. J. Chem.* **50**:1051–1064, 1972.
14. Young, J. C. Detection and determination of N-nitrosamines by thin-layer chromatography using fluorescamine. *J. Chromatogr.* **124**:17–28, 1976.
15. Ballweg, H. and Schmähl, D. Photolysis of nitrosamines. *Naturwissenschaften* **54**:116, 1967.
16. Chow, Y.-L. Photolysis of N-nitrosamines. *Tetrahedron Lett.* 2333–2338, 1964.
17. Doerr, R. C. and Fiddler, W. Photolysis of volatile nitrosamines at the picogram level as an aid to confirmation. *J. Chromatogr.* **140**:284–287, 1977.
18. Chuong, B. T. and Benarie, M. Method for determining N-nitrosamine in the atmosphere. *Sci. Total Environ.* **6**:181–193, 1976.
19. Eisenbrand, G. and Preussmann, R. A new method for the colorimetric determination of nitrosamines after cleavage of the N-nitroso group with hydrogen bromide in glacial acetic acid. *Arzneim.-Forsch.* **20**:1513–1517, 1970.
20. Johnson, E. M. and Walters, C. L. The specificity of the release of nitrite from N-nitrosamines by hydrobromic acid. *Anal. Lett.* **4**:383–386, 1971.
21. Garrett, E. R., Goto, S., and Stubbins, J. F. Kinetics of solvolyses of various N-alkyl-N-nitrosoureas in neutral and alkaline solutions. *J. Pharm. Sci.* **54**:119–123, 1965.
22. Preussmann, R. and Schaper-Druckrey, F. Investigation of a colorimetric procedure for determination of nitrosamides and comparison with other methods. In: *N-Nitroso Compounds—Analysis and Formation (Proc. Work Conf.)*: 81–86, Bogovski, E. A., Preussman, R., Walker, E. A., and Davis, W. (Eds.). IARC Sci. Publ. No. 3, Lyon, France, 1972.

23. Neale, S. Effect of pH and temperature on nitrosamide-induced mutation in *Escherichia coli. Mutat. Res.* **14**:155–164, 1972.
24. Veleminsky, J., Gichner, T., and Pokorny, V. The action of 1-alkyl-1-nitrosoureas and 1-alkyl-3-nitro-1-nitrosoguanidines on the M_1 generation of barley and *Arabidopsis thaliana* (L.) Heynh. *Biol. Plant.* **9**:249–262, 1967.
25. Frei, J. V. Toxicity, tissue changes, and tumor induction in inbred Swiss mice by methylnitrosamine and -amide compounds. *Cancer Res.* **30**:11–17, 1970.
26. Olah, G. A., Donovan, D. J., and Keefer, L. K. Carcinogen chemistry. I. Reactions of protonated dialkylnitrosamines leading to alkylating and aminoalkylating agents of potential metabolic significance. *J. Natl. Cancer Inst.* **54**:465–472, 1975.
27. Preussmann, R., Deutsch-Wenzel, R., and Eisenbrand, G. The effect of heavy metal ions on the rate of decomposition of N-ethyl-N-nitrosourea and other carcinogenic N-nitrosamides. *Z. Krebsforsch. Klin. Onkol.* **84**:75–80, 1975.
28. Kimmerman, F. K., Schwaier, R., and Laer, U. v. The influence of pH on the mutagenicity in yeast of N-methylnitrosamides and nitrous acid. *Z. Vererbungsl.* **97**:68–71, 1965.
29. Tempe, J., Heslot, H., and Morel, G. Study of the alkaline hydrolysis of some N-nitroso precursors of diazoalkanes. *C. R. Acad. Sci.* **258**:5470–5473, 1964.
30. Zahradnick, R. N-Nitroso derivatives of secondary amines. I. Kinetics and mechanism of the decomposition in strong acids. *Chem. Listy* **51**:937–945, 1957.
31. Emmons, W. D. and Ferris, A. F. Oxidation reactions with pertrifluoracetic acid. *J. Am. Chem. Soc.* **75**:4623–4624, 1953.
32. Emmons, W. D. Peroxytrifluoracetic acid. I. The oxidation of nitrosamines to nitramines. *J. Am. Chem. Soc.* **76**:3468–3470, 1954.
33. Telling, G. M. A gas-liquid chromatographic procedure for the detection of volatile N-nitrosamines at the ten parts per billion level in foodstuffs after conversion to their corresponding nitramines. *J. Chromatogr.* **73**:79–87, 1972.
34. Althorpe, J., Goddard, D. A., Sissons, D. J., and Telling, G. M. The gas chromatographic determination of nitrosamines at the picogram level by conversion to their corresponding nitramines. *J. Chromatogr.* **53**:371–373, 1970.
35. Toda, K., Izaki, Y., and Itokawa, T. Conditions for converting nitrosamines to nitramines. *Shokuhin Eiseigaku Zasshi* **14**:561–564, 1973.
36. Castegnaro, M., Pignatelli, B., and Walker, E. A. Investigation of the use of 2-butanone peroxide in oxidation of nitrosamines for gas chromatography. In: *N-Nitroso Compounds—Analysis and Formation (Proc. Work Conf.)*: 87–89, Bogovski, P., Preussmann, R., Walker, E. A., and Davis, W. (Eds.). IARC Sci. Publ. No. 3, Lyon, France, 1972.

37. Preussmann, R. The oxidative breakdown of nitrosamines by enzyme-free model systems. *Arzneim.-Forsch.* 14:769–774, 1964.

38. Chow, Y.-L. Photochemistry of nitroso compounds in solution. V. Photolysis of N-nitrosodialykylamines. *Can. J. Chem.* 45:53–62, 1967.

39. McCalla, D. R., Reuvers, A., and Kitai, R. Inactivation of biologically active N-methyl-N-nitroso compounds in aqueous solutions: effect of various conditions of pH and illumination. *Can. J. Biochem.* 46:807–811, 1968.

40. Crosby, N. T. Nitrosamines in foodstuffs. In: *Residue Reviews* 64: 88–93, Gunther, F. A. and Gunther, J. D. (Eds.). Springer-Verlag, New York, 1976.

41. Fridman, A. L., Mukhametshin, F. M., and Novikov, S. S. Advances in the chemistry of aliphatic N-nitrosamines. *Russ. Chem. Rev. (Engl. Transl.)* 40:34–50, 1971.

42. Preussmann, R. On the significance of N-nitroso compounds as carcinogens and on problems related to their chemical analysis. In: *N-Nitroso Compounds–Analysis and Formation (Proc. Work Conf.)*: 6–9, Bogovski, P., Preussmann, R., Walker, E. A., and Davis, W. (Eds.). IARC Sci. Publ. No. 3, Lyon, France, 1972.

43. Druckrey, H., Preussmann, R., Ivankovic, S., Schmähl, D., Afkham, J., Blum, G., Mennel, H. D., Müller, M., Petropoulos, P., and Schneider, H. Organotropic carcinogenic effects of 65 different N-nitroso compounds on BD-rats. *Z. Krebsforsch.* 69:103–201, 1967.

44. Veleminsky, J., Osterman-Golkar, S., and Ehrenberg, L. Reaction rates and biological action of N-methyl- and N-ethyl-N-nitrosourea. *Mutat. Res.* 10:169–174, 1970.

45. Magee, P. N. and Barnes, J. M. Carcinogenic nitroso compounds. In: *Advances in Cancer Research* 10:164–246, Haddow, A. and Weinhouse, S. (Eds.). Academic Press, New York, 1967.

46. Fine, D. H. and Rounbehler, D. P. Detection system with liquid chromatograph. *U.S. Patent #3,996,004.* Dec. 7, 1976.

47. White, E. H. The chemistry of the N-alkyl-N-nitrosamides. II. A new method for the deamination of aliphatic amines. *J. Am. Chem. Soc.* 77:6011–6014, 1955.

48. Tate, R. L. III and Alexander, M. Resistance of nitrosamines to microbial attack. *J. Environ. Qual.* 5:131–133, 1976.

49. Tate, R. L. III and Alexander, M. Stability of nitrosamines in samples of lake water, soil, and sewage. *J. Natl. Cancer Inst.* 54:327–330, 1975.

50. Rowland, I. R. and Grasso, P. The bacterial degradation of nitrosamines. *Biochem. Soc. Trans.* 3:185–188, 1975.

51. Mikhailovskii, N. Ya., Korolev, A. A., Il'nitskii, A. P., and Rumyantsev, P. G. Study of the barrier role of some water purification methods in relation to nitrosamines. In: *Kantserogennye N-Nitrozosoedineniya–Deistvie, Sint, Opred., Mater. Simp. N-Nitrozosoedineniyam, 2nd:* 86–88, Bogovskii, S. P. (Ed.). Inst. Eksp. Klin. Med., Tallinn, U.S.S.R., 1975.

52. Polo, J. and Chow, Y.-L. Efficient degradation of nitrosamines by photolysis. In: *Environmental N-Nitroso Compounds—Analysis and Formation (Proc. Work Conf.)*: 473–486, Walker, E. A., Bogovski, P., Griciute, L., and Davis, W. (Eds.). IARC Sci. Publ. No. 14, Lyon, France, 1976.
53. Feigl, F. and Anger, V. *Spot Tests in Organic Analysis:* 292–294, 586–587, 7th English ed., translated by Oesper, R. E. Elsevier, New York, 1975.
54. Williams, D. L. H. Alternative method for the decomposition of nitrosamines in solution. *Food Cosmet. Toxicol.* **13**:302, 1975.
55. Morimoto, K., Yamaha, T., Nakadate, M., and Suzuki, I. Chemical stability, alkylating activity, and lipophilicity of 1,1-ethylene-bis(1-nitrosourea) and related compounds. *Gann* **69**:139–142, 1978.
56. Jones, E. C. S. and Kenner, J. The analogy between the benzidine change and the dissociation of oxides of nitrogen. A new reagent for the recovery of secondary bases from nitrosamines and for purifying amines. *J. Chem. Soc.:* 711–715, 1932.

N-NITROSODIBUTYLAMINE* (924-16-3)

Degradation Technique	Remarks	Reference
Photo-decomposition	Photolysis in acidified, aqueous methanol gave butyraldehyde, dibutylamine, and dibutylamine monooxime.	1
Photo-decomposition Oxidation Reduction Hydrolysis	Sensitive to light, especially UV. Oxidized to the nitramine. Reduced to the corresponding hydrazine and/or amine. Is stable in the dark at neutral or alkaline pH; is less stable in acid. HBr readily splits it to give the amine and NOBr under anhydrous conditions.	2

*See also nitrosamines and nitrosamides.

N-Nitrosodibutylamine

1. Chow, Y.-L. Photolysis of N-nitrosamines. *Tetrahedron Lett.:* 2333–2338, 1964.
2. *Int. Agency Res. Cancer Monogr.* **4**:197, Lyon, France, 1974.

N-NITROSODIETHYLAMINE* (55-18-5)

Degradation Technique	Remarks	Reference
Photo-decomposition	A 1% aqueous solution was exposed to daylight until characteristic absorption maxima disappeared. Product was not carcinogenic for rats.	1
Photo-decomposition Oxidation Reduction Hydrolysis	Photochemically reactive, especially to UV. Oxidized by strong reagents to give corresponding nitramine. Reduced by various reagents to the corresponding hydrazine and/or amine. Hydrolyzed by HBr in HOAc. Stable at neutral or alkaline pH in the dark.	2
Oxidation	In vitro hydroxylation, using Fe^{+2} and ascorbic acid, produced a mutagen presumed to be the same as the metabolically-activated carcinogen.	3
Photo-decomposition	The photolysis of the vapor at $100°C$ was studied. Rupture of the N-N bond occurred. Products were identified.	4

*See also nitrosamines and nitrosamides.

N-Nitrosodiethylamine

1. Ballweg, H., Krüger, F. W., and Schmähl, D. Loss of carcinogenic action by photolyzed diethylnitrosamine. *Naturwissenschaften* 54:591, 1967.
2. *Int. Agency Res. Cancer Monogr.* 1:107, Lyon, France, 1972.
3. Malling, H. V. Mutagenicity of two potent carcinogens, dimethylnitrosamine and diethylnitrosamine, in *Neurospora crassa. Mutat. Res.* 3:537–540, 1966.
4. Bamford, C. H. A study of the photolysis of organic nitrogen compounds. Part I. Dimethyl- and diethyl-nitrosoamines. *J. Chem. Soc.:* 12–17, 1939.

N-NITROSODIMETHYLAMINE* (62-75-9)

Degradation Technique	Remarks	Reference
Photo-decomposition Chemical	The effects of pH variation and HNO_2-scavengers were tested using fluorescent and UV irradiation and $T_{1/2}$ determined. Possible dangerous products from reduction by Al in alkali or from HBr in other degradation procedures were mentioned	1
Photo-decomposition	Photolysis to form $(CH_3)_2 NH$, N_2, and $N_2 O$ was faster in acidic than in neutral or basic solutions. The effect of HNO_2-scavengers was studied.	2
Photo-decomposition	An ESR study showed that filtered Hg-lamp radiation (>300 nm) at $77°K$ resulted in N-N bond cleavage.	3
Photo-decomposition	Further ESR evidence was found for direct N-N cleavage of NDMA by filtered radiation from a high-pressure mercury lamp.	4
Photo-decomposition	^{14}C-NDMA lost its alkylating ability after exposure to daylight. No details.	5
Photo-decomposition	A study of NDMA loss from wastewater. The rate of evaporation was greater at higher pH's; the rate of photolysis by sunlight was greater at lower pH's.	6
Photo-decomposition	The photolysis of vapors of NDMA and NDEA was studied at $100°C$. Rupture of the N-N bond occurred. Products were identified.	7
Photo-decomposition	Irradiation of NDMA in air with UV lamps for 1 hr almost completely converted it to an unidentified compound plus NO, CO, and HCHO. Half of the NDMA in air was destroyed by sunlight in 0.5 hr.	8
Photo-decomposition Reduction	The procedures were not very efficient. An attempt was made to identify products.	9

*See also nitrosamines and nitrosamides.

N-NITROSODIMETHYLAMINE (62-75-9)
continued

Degradation Technique	Remarks	Reference
Ionizing radiation	Gamma radiation from ^{60}Co degraded NDMA to form NO_2^-, NO_3^-, CH_3NH_2, $(CH_3)_2NH$, and $(CH_3)_2NNO_2$.	10
Oxidation	Treatment with H_2O_2 and CF_3COOH produced dimethylnitramine, which was used as the basis for microanalysis by GLC.	11
Oxidation	*In vitro* hydroxylation, using Fe^{+2} and ascorbic acid, produced a mutagen for *Neurospora* presumed to be the same as the metabolically-activated carcinogen.	12
Oxidation	A commercial wet-air oxidation system was described for degrading the alkaline waste-water from the manufacture of 1,1-dimethylhydrazine. Oxidation was not significantly affected by pH or catalyst at $320°C$.	13
Thermal	The $T_{1/2}$ at $110°C$ was shortest at pH 5.5 and pH 8.5 (16 and 15 days, respectively). Included data for a few other nitrosamines.	14
Microbial	NDMA was stable for one month in manure and manure extracts under aerobic or anaerobic conditions at $25-30°C$, and in aerobic sewage effluents.	15
Microbial	Several bacterial species were able to degrade NDMA to the amine, but only slowly, at pH 7 and $37°C$. Diphenylnitrosamine was degraded somewhat more readily.	16
	Activated C efficiently removed NDMA from the alkaline waste produced in dimethylhydrazine production, but disposal of the adsorbent remained a problem.	17

NDEA: N-nitrosodiethylamine   NDMA: N-nitrosodimethylamine

N-Nitrosodimethylamine

1. Polo, J. and Chow, Y.-L. Efficient photolytic degradation of nitrosamines. *J. Natl. Cancer Inst.* **56**:997–1001, 1976.

2. Polo, J. and Chow, Y.-L. Efficient degradation of nitrosamines by photolysis. In: *Environmental N-Nitroso Compounds—Analysis and Formation (Proc. Work Conf.):* 473–486, Walker, E. A., Bogovski, P., Griciute, L., and Davis, W. (Eds.). IARC Sci. Publ. No. 14, Lyon, France, 1976.

3. Jakubowski, E. and Wan, J. K. S. ESR study of UV-irradiated dimethylnitrosamine at 77°K: evidence of the primary N-N cleavage. *Mol. Photochem.* **5**:439–441, 1973.

4. Adeleke, B. B. and Wan, J. K. S. Further ESR evidence of the primary N-N cleavage in the photolysis of dimethylnitrosamine: indirect spin trapping of the primary radical NO. *Mol. Photochem.* **6**:329–331, 1974.

5. Ballweg, H., Krüger, F. W., and Schmähl, D. Loss of carcinogenic action by photolyzed diethylnitrosamine. *Naturwissenschaften* **54**:591, 1967.

6. MacNaughton, M. G. and Stauffer, T. B. *The Evaporation and Degradation of N-Nitroso Dimethyl Amine in Aqueous Solutions.* U.S. NTIS AD Rep. **A020922**, 22 pp., Springfield, Virginia, 1975.

7. Bamford, C. H. A study of the photolysis of organic nitrogen compounds. Part I. Dimethyl- and diethyl-nitrosamines. *J. Chem. Soc.:* 12–17, 1939.

8. Hanst, P. L., Spence, J. W., and Miller, M. Atmospheric chemistry of N-nitroso dimethylamine. *Environ, Sci. Technol.* **11**:403–405, 1977.

9. Grilli, S., Tosi, M. R., and Prodi, G. Degradation of dimethylnitrosoamine catalysed by physical and chemical agents. *Gann* **66**:481–488, 1975.

10. Hirano, T. Effect of gamma irradiation on the decomposition of dimethylnitrosamine in aqueous solutions. *J. Tokyo Univ. Fish.* **59**:1–7, 1972.

11. Sen, N. P. Gas-liquid chromatographic determination of dimethylnitrosamine as dimethylnitramine at picogram levels. *J. Chromatogr.* **51**:301–304, 1970.

12. Malling, H. V. Mutagenicity of two potent carcinogens, dimethylnitrosamine and diethylnitrosamine, in *Neurospora crassa. Mutat. Res.* **3**:537–540, 1966.

13. Shelton, S. P. *NDMA Treatability Studies.* U.S. NTIS AD Rep. **A038658**, 15 pp., Springfield, Virginia, 1976.

14. Fan, T.-Y. and Tannenbaum, S. R. Stability of N-nitroso compounds. *J. Food Sci.* **37**:274–276, 1972.

15. Mosier, A. R. and Torbit, S. Synthesis and stability of dimethylnitrosamine in cattle manure. *J. Environ. Qual.* **5**:465–468, 1976.

16. Rowlan, I. R. and Grasso, P. Degradation of N-nitrosamines by intestinal bacteria. *Appl. Microbiol.* **29**:7–12, 1975.

17. MacNaughton, M. G. and Stauffer, T. B. *Treatment of N-nitrosodimethylamine contaminated waste with activated carbon.* U.S. NTIS AD Rep. **A039229**, 18 pp., Springfield, Virginia, 1976.

N-NITROSODIPROPYLAMINE* (621-64-7)

Degradation Technique	Remarks	Reference
Reduction	1,1-Dipropylhydrazine was formed in 41% and 60% yields by reducing it with LiAlH$_4$ and with Na in liquid NH$_3$, respectively. Care was necessary to prevent a delayed violent reaction when LiAlH$_4$ was used. Other nitrosamines were reduced by these procedures.	1

*See also nitrosamines and nitrosamides.

N-Nitrosodipropylamine

1. Zimmer, H., Audrieth, L. F., Zimmer, M., and Rowe, R. A. The synthesis of unsymmetrically disubstituted hydrazines. *J. Am. Chem. Soc.* 77:790–793, 1955.

1,4-DINITROSOPIPERAZINE* (140-79-4)

Degradation Technique	Remarks	Reference
Hydrolysis	Reacted with HBr in glacial HOAc to form HNO$_2$ in 90% yield in 15 min at room temperature.	1

*See also nitrosamines and nitrosamides.

1,4-Dinitrosopiperazine

1. Johnson, E. M. and Walters, C. L. The specificity of the release of nitrite from N-nitrosamines by hydrobromic acid. *Anal. Lett.* 4:383–386, 1971.

N-NITROSOPIPERIDINE* (100-75-4)

Degradation Technique	Remarks	Reference
Photo-decomposition	A flash photolysis study in dilute acid showed that a piperidinium radical formed which initiated elimination, reduction, and addition reactions.	1
Photo-decomposition	A kinetic study was made of the flash photolysis in dilute acid. The reactive transient formed was the piperidinium radical.	2
Photo-decomposition	Readily decomposed by photolysis in the presence of acid. Products were identified.	3
Photo-decomposition	The photolysis in acid was studied in detail in different solvents and at varied temperatures. Products were identified.	4
Reduction	Reduction with $LiAlH_4$ gave N-aminopiperidine.	5
Thermal	A study was made of thermal decomposition kinetics at 265-312°C.	6

*See also nitrosamines and nitrosamides.

N-Nitrosopiperidine

1. Lau, M. P., Cessna, A. J., Chow, Y.-L., and Yip, R. W. Flash photolysis of N-nitrosopiperidine. The reactive transient. *J. Am. Chem. Soc.* **93**:3808-3809, 1971.
2. Cessna, A. J., Sugamori, S. E., Yip, R. W., Lau, M. P., Snyder, R. S., and Chow, Y.-L. Flash photolysis studies of N-chloro- and N-nitrosopiperidine in aqueous solution. Assignment and reactivity of the piperidinium radical. *J. Am. Chem. Soc.* **99**:4044-4048, 1977.
3. Chow, Y.-L. Photochemistry of nitroso compounds in solution. V. Photolysis of N-nitrosodialkylamines. *Can. J. Chem.* **45**:53-62, 1967.
4. Chow, Y.-L. Photolysis of N-nitrosamines. *Tetrahedron Lett.:* 2333-2338, 1964.
5. Smith, P. A. S. and Kalenda, N. W. Investigation of some dialkylamino isocyanides. *J. Org. Chem.* **23**:1599-1603, 1958.
6. Golovanova, O. F., Pepekin, V. I., Korsunskii, B. L., Gafurov, R. G., Eremenko, L. T., and Dubovitskii, F. I. Kinetic and thermochemical studies of N-nitrosopiperidine. *Izv. Akad. Nauk SSSR, Ser. Khim.:* 1495-1497, 1974.

N-METHYL-N'-NITRO-N-NITROSOGUANIDINE* (70–25–7)

Degradation Technique	Remarks	Reference
Hydrolysis	The effects of pH, temperature, and buffer were studied.	1
Hydrolysis	At 37°C in citrate-phosphate buffer, $T_{1/2}$ varied with pH: $T_{1/2}$ was 40 hr at pH 5, 0.6 hr at pH 8.	2
Hydrolysis	Decomposition was greater in phosphate at pH 7.5 than in Tris at pH 9. Included data for N-ethyl- and N-propylnitronitrosoguanidines.	3
Hydrolysis	Mutagenesis was correlated with MNNG degradation at alkaline pH. The effects of pH, buffer concentration, and temperature were studied. Hydrolysis was complete in 1 hr in 0.05 M Tris-maleate buffer, pH 10.	4
Hydrolysis Photo-decomposition	Toxic diazomethane was produced in alkaline solutions. Sunlight converted the orange crystals to green with loss of nitrogen oxides.	5
Photo-decomposition	When a solution of MNNG was illuminated by 800 foot-candles at pH 6.8, $T_{1/2}$ was about 6 hr.	6
Photo-decomposition Physical	Wavelengths above 340 nm produced free radicals in a benzene solution and resulted in the conversion of MNNG to N-methyl-N'-nitroguanidine. Optimal, but slow, free radical formation occurred while stirring solutions between pH 3 and pH 6 at 4°C.	7
Physical	MNNG will detonate under high impact. May also explode when melted in a sealed capillary tube.	8
Reaction with primary amines Reaction with secondary amines	N-substituted-N'-nitroguanidines with N_2 formed in reaction with primary amines; secondary amines caused decomposition, but some also produced nitroguanidine derivatives.	9
Reaction with amines	A study was made of the relationship between possible structures of MNNG and reactivity, using ethylamine as a typical amine.	10

*See also nitrosamines and nitrosamides.

N-METHYL-N'-NITRO-N-NITROSOGUANIDINE   (70–25–7)
(continued)

Degradation Technique	Remarks	Reference
Reaction with amines	A study was made of the products obtained by the reaction of MNNG with aniline and other amines.	11
Reaction with cysteine	At pH 7.4, 30°C, $T_{1/2}$ was about 55 min in the absence of cysteine. When cysteine was present (1:1 ratio), $T_{1/2}$ was about 1 min. Included data with nitrosomethylurea.	12
Reaction with cysteine	Reaction products were identified.	13
Reaction with nucleophiles	Various buffers and thiols were tested. The reaction was most rapid at alkaline pH ± cysteine.	14
Reaction with nucleophiles	Reactions with various nucleophiles, including water, were determined at 25°C and 37°C. Data were also given for N-ethylnitronitroso-guanidine.	15
Reaction with nucleophiles	MNNG slowly methylated and deaminated nucleic acid bases and their derivatives at pH 5.5–6.	16
Thermal Hydrolysis Reaction with 99% HNO₃ Reaction with alkylamines	Melts at 118°C with decomposition. Decomposed to diazomethane (toxic gas) in alkaline solution. Reaction with 99% HNO_3 at –40°C formed methyl nitroguanidine nitrate, which was completely hydrolyzed by water. In reaction with alkylamines, the methylnitrosamine group was replaced by alkylamino groups with vigorous gas formation.	17

MNNG: N-methyl-N'-nitro-N-nitrosoguanidine

N-Methyl-N'-nitro-N-nitrosoguanidine

1. La Polla, J. P., Harris, C. M., and Vary, J. C. Properties of N-methyl-N'-nitro-N-nitrosoguanidine and its action on *Bacillus subtilis* transforming DNA. *Biochem. Biophys. Res. Commun.* 49:133–138,1972.

2. Süssmuth, R. and Lingens, F. The mode of action of 1-nitroso-3-nitro-1-methyl-guanidine (NNMG) in mutagenesis. IV. Stability of NNMG, the relationship between the mutation rate and uptake of mutagen by the cell, and the methylation of sulfhydryl groups are dependent on pH. *Z. Naturforsch., Teil B* **24**:903–910, 1969.

3. Haga, J. J., Russell, B. R., and Chapel, J. F. The kinetics of decomposition of N-alkyl derivatives of nitrosoguanidine. *Cancer Res.* **32**:2085, 1972.

4. Delic, V., Hopwood, D. A., and Friend, E. J. Mutagenesis by N-methyl-N'-nitro-N-nitrosoguanidine (NTG) in *Streptomyces coelicolor. Mutat. Res.* **9**:167–182, 1970.

5. McKay, A. F. A new method of preparation of diazomethane. *J. Am. Chem. Soc.* **70**:1974–1975, 1948.

6. McCalla, D. R. Mutation of the *Euglena* chloroplast system. The mechanism of bleaching by nitrosoguanidine and related compounds. *J. Protozool.* **14**: 480–482, 1967.

7. Nagata, C., Nakadate, M., Ioki, Y., and Imamura, A. Electron spin resonance study on the free radical production from N-methyl-N'-nitro-N-nitroso-guanidine. *Gann* **63**:471–481, 1972.

8. *Handbook of Reactive Chemical Hazards:* 317, Bretherick, L. (Ed.). CRC Press, Cleveland, Ohio, 1975.

9. McKay, A. F. The preparation of N-substituted-N'-nitrosoguanidines by the reaction of primary amines with N-alkyl-N-nitroso-N-nitroguanidines. *J. Am. Chem. Soc.* **71**:1968–1970, 1949.

10. Imamura, A. and Nagata, C. A. molecular orbital study on the chemical reactivity and biological activity of N-methyl-N'-nitro-N-nitrosoguanidine and some related compounds. *Gann* **65**:417–422, 1974.

11. Henry, R. A. The reaction of amines with N-methyl-N-nitroso-N'-nitro-guanidine. *J. Am. Chem. Soc.* **72**:3287–3289, 1950.

12. Wheeler, G. P. and Bowdon, B. J. Comparison of the effects of cysteine upon the decomposition of nitrosoureas and of 1-methyl-3-nitro-1-nitro-soguanidine. *Biochem. Pharmacol.* **21**:265–267, 1972.

13. Schulz, U. and McCalla, D. R. Reactions of cysteine with N-methyl-N-nitroso-*p*-toluenesulfonamide and N-methyl-N'-nitro-N-nitrosoguanidine. *Can. J. Chem.* **47**:2021–2027, 1969.

14. Lawley, P. D. and Thatcher, C. J. Methylation of deoxyribonucleic acid in cultured mammalian cells by N-methyl-N'-nitro-N-nitrosoguanidine. *Biochem. J.* **116**:693–707, 1970.

15. Osterman-Golkar, S. Reaction kinetics of N-methyl-N'-nitro-N-nitroso-guanidine and N-ethyl-N'-nitro-N-nitrosoguanidine. *Mutat. Res.* **24**:219–226, 1974.

16. Lingens, F., Rau, J., and Süssmuth, R. The mode of action of 1-nitroso-3-nitro-1-methyl-guanidine in mutagenesis. II. Products of the reaction of 1-nitroso-3-nitro-1-methyl-guanidine with nucleic acid bases, nucleosides, nucleoside phosphates, and homopolyribonucleic acids. *Z. Naturforsch., Teil B* **23**:1565–1570, 1968.

17. McKay, A. F. and Wright, G. F. Preparation and properties of N-methyl-N-nitroso-N'-nitroguanidine. J. Am. Chem. Soc. 69:3028–3030, 1947.

N-NITROSO-N-ETHYLUREA* (759-73-9)

Degradation Technique	Remarks	Reference
Hydrolysis	A study was made of the effect of pH on the mutation of *Drosophila melanogaster* caused by ENU. At $25°C$, ENU was less stable at pH 8 than at pH 6 or pH 6.9.	1
Hydrolysis	In physiological saline at $37°C$, $T_{1/2}$ was 150 min. When hydrolyzed in growth medium with serum, $T_{1/2}$ was 15 min..	2
Hydolysis	In phosphate buffer, pH 7.25, $37°C$, $T_{1/2}$ was 7.7 min.	3
Hydrolysis Photo-decomposition	In aqueous solution at $20°C$, pH ($T_{1/2}$, hr): 4(190), 6(31), 7(1.5), 8(0.1), 9($\sim$0.05). Alkaline pH produced diazoethane (toxic gas). ENU is sensitive to light and humidity.	4

ENU: N-nitroso-N-ethylurea

*See also nitrosamines and nitrosamides.

N-Nitroso-N-ethylurea

1. Corwin, H. O. and Hanratty, W. P. The effect of pH on N-alkylnitrosoamide mutagenesis in *Drosophila*. *Mutat. Res.* 14:325–330, 1972.
2. Knox, P. Carcinogenic nitrosamides and cell cultures. *Nature* 259:671–673, 1976.
3. Goth, R. and Rajewsky, M. F. Ethylation of nucleic acids by ethylnitro-sourea-1-^{14}C in the fetal and adult rat. *Cancer Res.* 32:1501–1502, 1972.
4. *Int. Agency Res. Cancer Monogr.* 1:135, Lyon, France, 1972.

N-NITROSO-N-METHYLUREA* (684–93–5)

Degradation Technique	Remarks	Reference
Thermal	Storage at 30°C may result in an explosion. Even at 20°C, an explosion occurred after six months.	1
Thermal	A bottle containing 100 g exploded when stored at room temperature.	2
Thermal Reaction with ethanol Hydrolysis	A violent reaction may occur above 20°C to form N_2, H_2O, and methyl isocyanate. Below 20°C, N_2, water and trimethylisocyanuric acid ester were gradually formed. Reacted with ethanol to produce CH_3OH, N_2, and allophanic acid ester. Diazomethane (toxic) is produced at alkaline pH.	3
Hydrolysis	$T_{1/2}$ determined in NaCl + Na citrate: 9 hr at 37°C, 0.9 hr at 56°C.	4
Hydrolysis	In cell growth medium containing serum at 37°C, $T_{1/2}$ was less than 15 min. Products were N_2, CH_3OH, and isocyanate.	5
Hydrolysis	At pH 7.4, 37°C, $T_{1/2}$ was about 12 min. This was not significantly affected by cysteine.	6
Hydrolysis	Products of hydrolysis were not teratogenic when injected into rat embryos in concentrations which for the parent compound gave 100% malformations. No details.	7
Hydrolysis	A study of the mechanism of base-induced decomposition. In several cases, the toxic diazomethane product was removed as formed by allowing it to methylate p-nitrobenzoic acid.	8
Hydrolysis Photo-decomposition	At 20°C, in aqueous solution, pH ($T_{1/2}$, hr): 4(125), 6(24), 7(1.2), 8(0.1), 9(0.03). Alkaline pH produced diazomethane (toxic gas). Is sensitive to humidity and light.	9

N-NITROSO-N-METHYLUREA (684-93-5)
(continued)

Degradation Technique	Remarks	Reference
Hydrolysis Reaction with amines	Boiling in water produced N_2, CH_3OH, and HNCO; boiling with an amine in water produced N-substituted ureas.	10
Reaction with aniline	The products were phenylurea and methylaniline.	11

*See also nitrosamines and nitrosamides.

N-Nitroso-N-methylurea

1. *Handbook of Reactive Chemical Hazards:* 317, Bretherick, L. (Ed.). CRC Press, Cleveland, Ohio, 1975.
2. Sparrow, A. H. Hazards of chemical carcinogens and mutagens. *Science* 181:700–701, 1973.
3. Clusius, K. and Endtinger, F. Reactions with N^{15}. XXXV. Spontaneous and alcoholic decomposition of nitrosomethylurea. *Helv. Chim. Acta* 43:2063–2066, 1960.
4. Rosenkranz, H. S., Rosenkranz, S., and Schmidt, R. M. Effects of nitrosomethylurea and nitrosomethylurethan on the physical chemical properties of DNA. *Biochim. Biophys. Acta* 195:262–265, 1969.
5. Knox, P. Carcinogenic nitrosamides and cell cultures. *Nature* 259:671–673, 1976.
6. Wheeler, G. P. and Bowdon, B. J. Comparison of the effects of cysteine upon the decomposition of nitrosoureas and of 1-methyl-3-nitro-1-nitrosoguanidine. *Biochem. Pharmacol.* 21:265–267, 1972.
7. Miller, L. R. Teratogenicity of degradation products of 1-methyl-1-nitrosourea. *Anat. Rec.* 169:379–380, 1971.
8. Hecht, S. M. and Kozarich, J. W. Mechanism of the base-induced decomposition of N-nitroso-N-methylurea. *J. Org. Chem.* 38:1821–1824, 1973.
9. *Int. Agency Res. Cancer Monogr.* 1:125, Lyon, France, 1972.
10. Boivin, J. L. and Boivin, P. A. Preparation of N-substituted ureas from nitrosomethylureas. *Can. J. Chem.* 29:478–481, 1951.
11. Henry, R. A. The reaction of amines with N-methyl-N-nitroso-N'-nitroguanidine. *J. Am. Chem. Soc.* 72:3287–3289, 1950.

N-NITROSO-N-ETHYLURETHANE* (614-95-9)

Degradation Technique	Remarks	Reference
Reaction with thiols	Reacted at pH 7–7.5 to give N_2 and mixtures of other products, some of which were identified.	1
Photo-decomposition	Exposure of 30% aqueous ethanol solutions to sunshine or UV produced diethyltetrazodicar-boxylic acid.	2

*See also nitrosamines and nitrosamides.

N-Nitroso-N-ethylurethane

1. Schoental, R. and Rive, D. J. Interaction of N-alkyl-N-nitrosourethanes with thiols. *Biochem. J.* **97**:466–474, 1965.
2. Schoental, R. Photodecomposition of N-alkyl-N-nitroso-urethanes. *Nature* **198**:1089, 1963.

N-NITROSO-N-METHYLURETHANE* (615-53-2)

Degradation Technique	Remarks	Reference
Thermal	May explode if stored at >15°C. Explodes if distilled at atmospheric pressure.	1
Photo-decomposition Thermal Reaction with thiols Hydrolysis	Unstable: sensitive to light, may decompose upon heating. Highly reactive, especially with thiol groups. Alkaline pH produces diazomethane (toxic gas).	2
Photo-decomposition Thermal Hydrolysis Reduction	Exposure of an aqueous solution to light gave an acid reaction, indicating degradation. Decomposed when heated at atmospheric pressure. Reaction of an aqueous solution with NH_3 in the cold produced N_2, CH_3OH, and urethane. Reduction with Zn and HOAc apparently produced the corresponding hydrazine, but it was not isolated.	3

N-NITROSO-N-METHYLURETHANE (615-53-2)
(continued)

Degradation Technique	Remarks	Reference
Hydrolysis	$T_{1/2}$ determined in buffered, dilute ethanol at $37°C$: from about 77 hr at pH 6.05 to 2.3 min at pH 9.9. Data were included for N-methyl-N'-nitro-N-nitrosoguanidine.	4
Hydrolysis	$T_{1/2}$ determined in NaCl + Na citrate: 42.5 hr at $37°C$, 5.5 hr at $56°C$.	5
Photo-decomposition	Exposure of 10% aqueous ethanol solutions to sunshine or a UV lamp produced dimethyl-tetrazodicarboxylic acid and other unidentified products.	6
Reaction with thiols	Reacted at pH 6–7.5 to give N_2 and mixtures of other products, some of which were identified.	7
Reaction with cysteine	Among the products formed with cysteine, the esters were unstable at room temperature even at pH 7.	8

*See also nitrosamines and nitrosamides.

N-Nitroso-N-methylurethane

1. *Handbook of Reactive Chemical Hazards:* 406, Bretherick, L. (Ed.). CRC Press, Cleveland, Ohio, 1975.
2. *Int. Agency Res. Cancer Monogr.* 4:212, Lyon, France, 1974.
3. Klobbie, M. E. A. Action of nitrous acid on nitrogen compounds. *Recl. Trav. Chim. Pays-Bas* 9:134–154, 1890.
4. Lawley, P. D. Methylation of DNA by N-methyl-N-nitrosourethane and N-methyl-N-nitroso-N'-nitroguanidine. *Nature* 218:580–581, 1968.
5. Rosenkranz, H. S., Rosenkranz, S., and Schmidt, R. M. Effects of nitroso-methylurea and nitrosomethylurethan on the physical chemical properties of DNA. *Biochim. Biophys. Acta* 195:262–265, 1969.
6. Schoental, R. Photodecomposition of N-alkyl-N-nitroso-urethanes. *Nature* 198:1089, 1963.
7. Schoental, R. and Rive, D. J. Interaction of N-alkyl-N-nitrosourethanes with thiols. *Biochem. J.* 97:466–474, 1965.
8. Schoental, R. Instability of some of the products formed by the action of N-methyl-N-nitrosourethane on cysteine *in vitro*. Role of neighbouring groups in enzymatic and carcinogenic action. *Nature* 209:148–151, 1966.

CHLOROMETHYL ETHERS

BIS(CHLOROMETHYL)ETHER* (542-88-1)

Degradation Technique	Remarks	Reference
Hydrolysis	In the vapor phase, $T_{1/2}$ was 20 hr in a glass reactor at 20°C, 67% R.H.	1
Hydrolysis	The rate constants were determined in solutions of NaOH, HCl, and water at three temperatures.	2
Hydrolysis	BCME vapor was stable in air at 10 and 100 ppm at 70% R.H., 25°C, for at least 18 hr.	3
Hydrolysis	The hydrolyses of BCME and five related compounds were studied in water: dimethylformamide (3:1) at pH 7, 0°C. HCHO and 2HCl were produced and the $T_{1/2}$ for BCME was less than 2 min.	4
Hydrolysis	At 25°C in an aqueous solution of an anion-exchange resin, $T_{1/2}$ was about 1 min.	5
Hydrolysis	The rate of hydrolysis of BCME vapor varied with the stirring rate.	6
Hydrolysis	Hydrolysis yielded HCl and HCHO. No details.	7
Hydrolysis Reaction with 4-(p-nitrobenzyl)-pyridine	In 2 min, 70% of the BCME was hydrolyzed in D_2O, but 20% remained after 18 hr due to an equilibrium between the BCME and its products. In reaction with 4-(p-nitrobenzyl)-pyridine, a 60–75% yield of bis[4-(p-nitrobenzyl)-pyridinium chloride] was obtained overnight in acetone at room temperature.	8
Hydrolysis Reaction with NH_3	In homogeneous media (e.g., 50% CH_3OH/H_2O), hydrolysis to HCHO and HCl was rapidly catalyzed by alkali at 25°C. In the vapor phase, hydrolysis was also rapid when contaminated air	9

*See also aliphatic halides.

BIS(CHLOROMETHYL)ETHER (542-88-1)
(continued)

Degradation Technique	Remarks	Reference
	was scrubbed with a solution of 0.1% Na_2CO_3. Reaction with aqueous 1% NH_3 caused a rapid decomposition to hexamethylenetetramine.	
Oxidation	The flash point is less than $19°C$.	10
Photo-decomposition	$T_{1/2}$ was about 1 min in gas mixtures containing Cl_2 at $40°C$.	11
Chemical Thermal	A review, with 423 references, describing many displacement reactions, other chemical reactions, and the thermal decomposition of a large number of α-haloalkyl ethers.	12

BCME: bis(chloromethyl)ether

Bis(chloromethyl)ether

1. Tou, J. C. and Kallos, G. J. Kinetic study of the stabilities of chloromethyl methyl ether and bis(chloromethyl)ether in humid air. *Anal. Chem.* 46: 1866–1869, 1974.
2. Tou, J. C., Westover, L. B., and Sonnabend, L. F. Kinetic studies of bis-(chloromethyl)ether hydrolysis by mass spectrometry. *J. Phys. Chem.* 78: 1096–1098, 1974.
3. Nichols, R. W. and Merritt, R. F. Relative solvolytic reactivities of chloromethyl methyl ether and bis(chloromethyl)ether. *J. Natl. Cancer Inst.* 50: 1373–1374, 1973.
4. Van Duuren, B. L., Katz, C., Goldschmidt, B. M., Frenkel, K., and Sivak, A. Carcinogencity of halo-ethers. II. Structure-activity relationships of analogs of bis(chloromethyl)ether. *J. Natl. Cancer Inst.* 48:1431–1439, 1972.
5. Tou, J. C., Westover, L. B., and Sonnabend, L. F. Analysis of a non-cross-linked, water soluble anion exchange resin for the possible presence of parts per billion level of bis(chloromethyl)ether. *J. Am. Ind. Hyg. Assoc.* 36:374–378, 1975.
6. Tou, J. C. and Kallos, G. J. Possible formation of bis(chloromethyl)ether from the reactions of formaldehyde and chloride ion. *Anal. Chem.* 48:958–963, 1976.

7. Nelson, N. The chloroethers-occupational carcinogens: a summary of laboratory and epidemiology studies. *Ann. N.Y. Acad. Sci.* 271:81–90, 1976.

8. Van Duuren, B. L., Sivak, A., Goldschmidt, B. M., Katz, C., and Melchionne, S. Carcinogenicity of halo-ethers. *J. Natl. Cancer Inst.* 43:481–486, 1969.

9. Alvarez, M. and Rosen, R. T. Formation and decompositon of bis(chloromethyl)ether in aqueous media. *Int. J. Environ. Anal. Chem.* 4:241–246, 1976.

10. *Handbook of Reactive Chemical Hazards:* 304, Bretherick, L. (Ed.). CRC Press, Cleveland, Ohio, 1975.

11. Kallos, G. J. and Tou, J. C. Study of photolytic oxidation and chlorination reactions of dimethyl ether and chlorine in ambient air. *Environ. Sci. Technol.* 11:1101–1105, 1977.

12. Summers, L. The α-haloalkyl ethers. *Chem. Rev.* 55:301–353, 1955.

CHLOROMETHYL METHYL ETHER* (107-30-2)

Degradation Technique	Remarks	Reference
Hydrolysis	The effects of temperature, humidity, and reactor surface material were studied. $T_{1/2}$ was 5.8 min in the vapor phase in a glass reactor at 25°C, 60% R. H. Included data on bis(chloromethyl)ether.	1
Hydrolysis	In the vapor phase (25°C, 70% R. H.), $T_{1/2}$ was 6 min at 100 ppm; 3.5 min at 1000 ppm.	2
Hydrolysis	In water: dimethylformamide (3:1) at pH 7, 0°C, $T_{1/2}$ was less than 2 min. HCHO and HCl formed.	3
Hydrolysis	HCl, CH_3OH, and HCHO were products. No details.	4
Hydrolysis	A study of the hydrolysis in mixtures of acetone and water. LiBr increased the rate of hydrolysis.	5
Hydrolysis	Very rapid to yield HCHO, HCl, and CH_3OH. No details.	6
Solvolysis	A kinetic study of the solvolysis in various solvents at about 25°C. Rate constants were determined.	7

*See also aliphatic halides.

CHLOROMETHYL METHYL ETHER (107–30–2)
(continued)

Degradation Technique	Remarks	Reference
Oxidation	Flash point is less than 23°C.	8
Chemical Thermal	A review, with 423 references, describing many displacement reactions, and the thermal decomposition of a large number of α-haloalkyl ethers.	9

Chloromethyl methyl ether

1. Tou, J. C. and Kallos, G. J. Kinetic study of the stabilities of chloromethyl methyl ether and bis(chloromethyl)ether in humid air. *Anal. Chem.* **46**:1866–1869, 1974.
2. Nichols, R. W. and Merritt, R. F. Relative solvolytic reactivities of chloromethyl ether and bis(chloromethyl)ether. *J. Natl. Cancer Inst.* **50**:1373–1374, 1973.
3. Van Duuren, B. L., Katz, C., Goldschmidt, B. M., Frenkel, K., and Sivak, A. Carcinogenicity of halo-ethers. II. Structure-activity relationships of analogs of bis(chloromethyl)ether. *J. Natl. Cancer Inst.* **48**:1431–1439, 1972.
4. Nelson, N. The chloroethers-occupational carcinogens: a summary of laboratory and epidemiology studies. *Ann. N.Y. Acad. Sci.* **271**:81–90, 1976.
5. Ribar, T. and Glavas, M. Hydrolysis of monochlorodimethyl ether and its homologs. *Glas. Hem. Drus., Beograd.* **33**:517–521, 1968.
6. Van Duuren, B. L., Sivak, A., Goldschmidt, B. M., Katz, C., and Melchionne, S. Carcinogenicity of halo-ethers. *J. Natl. Cancer Inst.* **43**:481–486, 1969.
7. Jones, T. C. and Thornton, E. R. Solvolysis mechanisms. SN1-like behavior of methyl chloromethyl ether. Sensitivity to solvent ionizing power and α-deuterium isotope effect. *J. Am. Chem. Soc.* **89**:4863–4867, 1967.
8. *Handbook of Reactive Chemical Hazards:* 312, Bretherick, L. (Ed.). CRC Press, Cleveland, Ohio, 1975.
9. Summers, L. The α-haloalkyl ethers. *Chem. Rev.* **55**:301–353, 1955.

AMINOFLOURENE DERIVATIVES

N-ACETOXY-2-FLUORENYLACETAMIDE (6098–44–8)

Degradation Technique	Remarks	Reference
Reaction with nucleophiles	Reacted with methionine, RNA, and guanosine at 37°C. Products were identified.	1
Reaction with nucleophiles	Decolorized 2, 2-diphenyl-1-picrylhydrazyl almost completely in 4 hr at 45°C. Reacted with guanosine to a greater extent than with adenosine.	2
Hydrolysis Reaction with nucleophiles	The acetoxy group was removed completely in 1 hr at 25°C in 0.1 M NaOH. Kinetic studies were made for reactions with methionine and guanosine under varied conditions of buffer and acetone concentration.	3
Reaction with guanosine	Reacted readily at pH 7 in dilute ethanol at 37°C to form 8-(N-2-fluorenylacetamido) guanosine, which was hydrolyzed with HCl to give 8-(N-2-fluorenylamino) guanine. Toxicity of the products was not discussed except in the context of nucleic acid modification.	4
Reaction with methionine Thermal	Reacted at various pH's at 37°C to give partial conversion to 3-CH_3S-2-AAF. Toxicity not mentioned. N-acetoxy-2-AAF melts at 109–111°C, with decomposition.	5
Isomerization	N-(3-Acetoxy)-2-AAF was formed by acid catalysis during TLC on silica gel.	6
Isomerization	Incubation for 2 hr at 37°C in phosphate, pH 7.4, produced N-(1-acetoxy)-2-AAF as the main product. Other 2-AAF derivatives included in study.	7

2-AAF: N-2-fluorenylacetamide

N-Acetoxy-2-fluorenylacetamide

1. Yost, Y., Gutmann, H. R., and Rydell, R. E. The carcinogenicity of fluo-renylhydroxamic acids and N-acetoxy-N-fluorenylacetamides for the rat as related to the reactivity of the esters toward nucleophiles. *Cancer Res.* **35**: 447–459, 1975.
2. Scribner, J. D. and Naimy, N. K. Reactions of esters of N-hydroxy-2-acetam-idophenanthrene with cellular nucleophiles and the formation of free radicals upon decomposition of N-acetoxy-N-aryl-acetamides. *Cancer Res.* **33**:1159–1164, 1973.
3. Scribner, J. D., Miller, J. A., and Miller, E. C. Nucleophilic substitution on carcinogenic N-acetoxy-N-arylacetamides. *Cancer Res.* **30**:1570–1579, 1970.
4. Kriek, E., Miller, J. A., Juhl, U., and Miller, E. C. 8-(N-2-Fluorenyl-acetam-ido) guanosine, an arylamidation reaction product of guanosine and the carcinognen N-acetoxy-N-2-fluorenylacetamide in neutral solution. *Bio-chemistry* **6**:177–182, 1967.
5. Lotlikar, P. D., Scribner, J. D., Miller, J. A., and Miller, E. C. Reaction of esters of aromatic N-hydroxy amines and amides with methionine *in vitro:* a model for *in vivo* binding of amine carcinogens to protein. *Life Sci.* **5**: 1263–1269, 1966.
6. Yost, Y. and Gutmann, H. R. Hindered N-arylhydroxamic acids from aryl-amines *via* nitroso-compounds. *J. Chem. Soc.* **(C)**:2497–2499, 1970.
7. Gutmann, H. R., Malejka-Giganti, D., and McIver, R. Identification of car-cinogenic acetates of fluorenylhydroxamic acids by high-pressure liquid chromatography. *J. Chromatogr.* **115**:71–78, 1975.

N-2-FLUORENYLACETAMIDE (53–96–3)

Degradation Technique	Remarks	Reference
Oxidation	Filters, activated carbon, and polymeric adsorbents reduced the 2-AAF content of wastewater to the 0.2 ppb level. Contaminated filters and carbon were destroyed by incineration at 900°C.	1
Hydrolysis	2-Aminofluorene was obtained when 2-AAF was heated at 85°C for 2 hr in a methanolic solution of HCl. Basis for analysis.	2

2-AAF: N-2-fluorenylacetamide

N-2-Fluorenylacetamide

1. Nony, C. R., Treglown, E. J., and Bowman, M. C. Removal of trace levels of 2-acetylaminofluorene (2-AAF) from wastewater. *Sci. Total Environ.* 4:155–163, 1975.
2. Bowman, M. C. and King, J. R. Analysis of 2-acetylaminofluorene: residues in laboratory chow and microbiological media. *Biochem. Med.* 9:390–401, 1974.

AZIRIDINES

AZIRIDINES*

Degradation Technique	Remarks	Reference
Physico-chemical	Physical and chemical properties were given. Many reactions were described that may have practical value.	1
Physico-chemical	An excellent article giving properties, reactions, uses, etc., up to 1969.	2
Hydrolysis	2,2-Dimethylaziridine derivatives were stable at alkaline pH, but were hydrolyzed rapidly at pH 6 or pH 5. Unsubstituted aziridine derivatives were more slowly hydrolyzed.	3
Hydrolysis	2,2-Dimethylaziridine derivatives were stable for 3 hr at pH 10.8, but were very unstable at pH 5 at 25°C.	4
Hydrolysis	A kinetic study of the acid hydrolysis of aziridine, 2-methylaziridine, and 2,2-dimethyl-aziridine.	5
Reaction with γ-(4-nitroben-zyl)-pyridine	Heated for 20 min at pH 4–5 in a boiling water bath. Basis for colorimetric analysis.	6
Reduction	Hydrogenolysis over a Raney Ni catalyst at 25°C gave α- and β-amines.	7
Hydrolysis Reaction with nucleophiles	Rate constants for four aziridines were determined at 25°C with $HClO_4$ as catalyst. Rate constants were also measured for three of the aziridines at several temperatures at atmospheric pressure, and at 21°C at 8000 psi. Rate constants were determined for the reaction of four aziridines with seven nucleophiles at 25°C.	8
Reaction with amines	α,β-Diamines were formed in 55–68% yields when aziridines were reacted with amines in liquid NH_3 in the presence of NH_4Cl at elevated temperature and pressure.	9

*See also specific compounds.

Aziridines

1. Dermer, O. C. and Hart, A. W. Cyclic imines. In: *Kirk-Othmer: Encyclopedia of Chemical Technology, 2nd ed.* 11:526–548. John Wiley & Sons, New York, 1966.
2. Dermer, O. C. and Ham, G. E. *Ethylenimine and Other Aziridines.* Academic Press, New York, 1969.
3. Lalka, D. and Bardos, T. J. Reactions of 2,2-dimethylaziridine-type alkylating agents in biological systems. I. Colorimetric estimation and stability in physiological media. *J. Pharm. Sci.* 62:1294–1298, 1973.
4. Lalka, D., Jusko, W. J., and Bardos, T. J. Reactions of 2,2-dimethylaziridine-type alkylating agents in biological systems. II. Comparative pharmacokinetics in dogs. *J. Pharm. Sci.* 64:230–235, 1975.
5. Bunnett, J. F., McDonald, R. L., and Olsen, F. P. Kinetics of hydrolysis of aziridines in moderately concentrated mineral acids. Relationship of ϕ parameters to reaction mechanism. *J. Am. Chem. Soc.* 96:2855–2861, 1974.
6. Epstein, J., Rosenthal, R. W., and Ess, R. J. Use of γ-(4-nitrobenzyl)pyridine as analytical reagent for ethylenimines and alkylating agents. *Anal. Chem.* 27:1435–1439, 1955.
7. Sugi, Y., Nagata, M., and Mitsui, S. The catalytic hydrogenolysis of alkyl-substituted aziridines. *Bull. Chem. Soc. Jpn.* 48:1663–1664, 1975.
8. Earley, J. E., O'Rourke, C. E., Clapp, L. B., Edwards, J. O., and Lawes, B. C. Reactions of ethylenimines. IX. The mechanisms of ring openings of ethylenimines in acidic aqueous solutions. *J. Am. Chem. Soc.* 80:3458–3462, 1958.
9. Clapp, L. B. Reactions of ethylenimines: with ammonia and amines. *J. Am. Chem. Soc.* 70:184–186, 1948.

DIMETHYLETHYLENIMINE* (2658-24-4: 2,2-ISOMER)

Degradation Technique	Remarks	Reference
Reduction	Hydrogenolysis of the 2,2-isomer over a Raney Ni catalyst at 25°C gave mostly the β-amine. 67% reduction occurred in 30 min.	1
Reduction	*tert*-Butylamine was produced in 75–82% yield by hydrogenation of the 2,2-isomer over Raney Ni. Reaction time was about 2 hr at 40–60 psi, 10–15 min at 3000 psi.	2

*See also aziridines.

Dimethylethylenimine

1. Sugi, Y., Nagata, M., and Mitsui, S. The catalytic hydrogenolysis of alkyl-substituted aziridines. *Bull. Chem. Soc. Jpn.* 48:1663–1664, 1975.
2. Campbell, K.N., Sommers, A. H., and Campbell, B. K. *tert*-Butylamine. In: *Organic Syntheses:* 12–15, Shriner, R. L. (Ed.). John Wiley & Sons, New York, 1947.

ETHYLENIMINE* (151–56–4)

Degradation Technique	Remarks	Reference
Hydrolysis	Rapid degradation to ethanolamine occurred in saturated phosphate buffer at pH 9. Included data on other aziridine insect sterilants.	1
Hydrolysis	Very slow hydrolysis occurred at pH 6, pH 7, or pH 8 in phosphate buffer at 27°C.	2
Hydrolysis Oxidation	Heating for 30 min at 100°C yielded ethanolamine. Addition of $NaHCO_3$ and $NaIO_4$ oxidized the ethanolamine to HCHO when heated for 30 min at 40°C. Basis for analysis.	3
Oxidation Polymerization	Flash point: –11°C. Exothermic polymerization, catalyzed by aqueous acids, may be violent unless controlled (dilution, slow addition, cooling). Polymerization by CO_2 minimized by storing over Na or K.	4
Polymerization Reaction with nucleophiles	Traces of acid catalyzed the formation of water-soluble polyethylenimine. Formed many aminoethylated derivatives by nucleophilic attack. No details.	5
Reaction with nucleophiles	A very rapid reaction occurred at 20°C with several nucleophilic vinyl derivatives.	6
Reaction with glutathione	A kinetic study of the aminoethylation of glutathione at pH 8.6 with an excess of ethylenimine.	7
Reaction with 4-(*p*-nitroben-zyl)-pyridine	A rapid reaction occurred at 50°C. Other aziridine derivatives reacted more slowly.	8

*See also aziridines.

ETHYLENIMINE (151-56-4)
(continued)

Degradation Technique	Remarks	Reference
Photo-decomposition	The products of ethylenimine vapor degradation were determined under various conditions of irradiation using a Kr or Xe lamp.	9
Photo-decomposition	The products of UV and of gamma irradiation of ethylenimine vapor were determined.	10
Chemical	A few hazardous reactions were cited.	11
Reaction with amines	The heterocyclic ring was split by the addition of primary or secondary amines in the presence of $AlCl_3$. The exothermic reactions were controlled by placing the reaction flask in an ice-bath.	12

Ethylenimine

1. Beroza, M. and Borkovec, A. B. The stability of tepa and other aziridine chemosterilants. *J. Med. Chem.* 7:44–49, 1964.
2. Pomonis, J. G., Severson, R. F., Hermes, P. A., Zaylskie, R. G., and Terranova, A. C. Analysis of insect chemosterilants. Action of phosphate buffers on aziridine. *Anal. Chem.* 43:1709–1712, 1971.
3. Salyamon, G. S. and Popelkovskaya, M. V. Determination of ethylenimine in the air. *Gig. Sanit.* 37(3):117–118, 1972.
4. *Handbook of Reactive Chemical Hazards:* 314, Bretherick, L. (Ed.). CRC Press, Cleveland, Ohio, 1975.
5. Fishbein, L., Flamm, W. G., and Falk, H. L. *Chemical Mutagens:* 143–145. Academic Press, New York, 1970.
6. Dore, J. C. and Viel, C. Research on antitumor chemotherapy. XII. Correlation between ethylenimine addition and cytotoxic properties on tumor cells of compounds with activated ethylene double bonds. *Eur. J. Med. Chem.-Chim. Ther.* 9:666–672, 1974.
7. Raftery, M. A. and Cole, R. D. On the aminoethylation of proteins. *J. Biol. Chem.* 241:3457–3461, 1966.
8. Lalka, D. and Bardos, T. J. Cyclophosphamide, 2,2-dimethylaziridines and other alkylating agents as inhibitors of serum cholinesterase. *Biochem. Pharmacol.* 24:455–462, 1975.

9. Kawasaki, M., Iwasaki, M., Ibuki, T., and Takezaki. Y. Primary processes of the photolysis of ethylenimine at Xe and Kr resonance lines. *J. Chem. Phys.* **59**:6321–6327, 1973.
10. Scala, A. A. and Salomon, D. The gas phase photolysis and γ radiolysis of ethylenimine. *J. Chem. Phys.* **65**:4455–4461, 1976.
11. *Hazards in the Chemical Laboratory, 2nd ed.:* 144, Muir, G. D. (Ed.). The Chemical Society, London, 1977.
12. Hicks, Z. A. and Coleman, G. H. The addition of amines to ethylenimine. *Proc. Iowa Acad. Sci.* **53**:207–209, 1946.

PROPYLENIMINE* (75-55-8)

Degradation Technique	Remarks	Reference
Oxidation	Flash point: $-10°C$.	1
Chemical	Flammable. Polymerized easily. Hydrolysis produced methylethanolamine. Reacted with carbonyl compounds, quinones, and sulfonyl halides. No details.	2
Reduction	Hydrogenolysis over a Raney Ni catalyst at $25°C$ gave 87% β- and 13% α-amine.	3

*See also aziridines.

Propylenimine

1. *Handbook of Reactive Chemical Hazards:* 369, Bretherick, L. (Ed.). CRC Press, Cleveland, Ohio, 1975.
2. *Int. Agency Res. Cancer Monogr.* **9**:61, Lyon, France, 1975.
3. Sugi, Y., Nagata, M., and Mitsui, S. The catalytic hydrogenolysis of alkyl-substituted aziridines. *Bull. Chem. Soc. Jpn.* **48**:1663–1664, 1975.

AROMATIC AMINES AND
RELATED COMPOUNDS

4-AMINOBIPHENYL (92-67-1)

Degradation Technique	Remarks	Reference
Oxidation Diazotization Acetylation Alkylation	Oxidized by air. No other details given.	1
Oxidation	Primary aromatic amines were oxidized by nitrosodisulfonate. The toxicity of the reagent and products was not discussed.	2
Oxidation	Peracetic acid oxidation yielded 4,4'-azobis-biphenyl and 4-nitrobiphenyl.	3
Deamination	Biphenyl was obtained in 33% yield when 4-aminobiphenyl was deaminated by treatment with $H(H_2PO_2)$ and $NaNO_2$.	4

4-Aminobiphenyl

1. *Int. Agency Res. Cancer Monogr.* 1:74, Lyon, France, 1972.
2. Teuber, H.-J. and Jellinek, G. Reactions with nitrosodisulfonate. VII. Oxidation of primary aromatic amines. *Chem. Ber.* 87:1841–1848, 1954.
3. Gutmann, H. R. The oxidation of N-2-fluorenamine and 4-aminobiphenyl by peracetic acid. *Experientia* 20:128–129, 1964.
4. Henry, R. A. and Finnegan, W. G. An improved procedure for the deamination of 5-aminotetrazole. *J. Am. Chem. Soc.* 76:290–291, 1954.

4-NITROBIPHENYL (92-93-3)

Degradation Technique	Remarks	Reference
Reduction	Can be reduced to 4-aminobiphenyl; no details.	1
Oxidation	Prolonged warming with powdered KOH in benzene produced $3\text{-}OH\text{-}4\text{-}NO_2$-biphenyl; no details.	

4-Nitrobiphenyl

1. *Int. Agency Res. Cancer Monogr.* 4:113, Lyon, France, 1974.

BENZIDINE (92-87-5)

Degradation Technique	Remarks	Reference
Diazotization	Bis(diazodiphenyl) chloride was the product formed during the decontamination of wastewater. However, excess $NaNO_2$ was present in the discharge.	1
Chemical	No details given. Mentioned diazotization, oxidation, acetylation, and alkylation.	2
Chemical	Many reactions were described that may have useful applications.	3
Chemical	Standard reactions of primary aromatic amines were described: oxidation with chloramine-T or NaOCl; diazotization with $NaNO_2$ and coupling with 2,3-hydroxynaphthoic acid or R-salt; reaction with 1,2-naphthoquinone-4-sulfonate. Bases for analyses.	4
Reaction with dialkyl acetylenedicarboxylates	The addition of dialkyl acetylenedicarboxylates to carcinogenic amines was described. Benzidine gave 91% yield of product, which was to be tested for carcinogenicity.	5
Microwave discharge	AgCl catalyzed the degradation to NH_4Cl in the presence of H_2 at 45 MHz.	6
Oxidation	Darkened on exposure to air and light.	7

BENZIDINE (92-87-5)
(continued)

Degradation Technique	Remarks	Reference
Oxidation	Iodide catalyzed the oxidation by H_2O_2.	8
Oxidation	Mn^{+3} was used for the oxidation, which produced the quinone diimine.	9
Oxidation	The mechanism of oxidation by Mn^{+3} was further studied.	10
Oxidation	A hemin-imidazole complex catalyzed the oxidation by H_2O_2.	11
Oxidation	A kinetic study of the oxidation by H_2O_2, catalyzed by Cr ions.	12
Oxidation	A solution of 2.5% NaOCl was recommended for decontaminating work clothes.	13
Oxidation	A kinetic study of the oxidation by periodate as catalyzed by Ru ions.	14
Oxidation	The effect of pH was included in this study of oxidation by periodate and Ru ions.	15
Oxidation	A study of semiquinone formation during the oxidation with $Ce(SO_4)_2$ and Br_2 at pH 0-9.	16
Oxidation	$Co(ClO_4)_3$ produced the quinonediimine without any semiquinone.	17
Oxidation	Hydrated MnO_2 produced the quinonediimine quantitatively in HCl at room temperature.	18
Oxidation	Oxidation by H_2O_2 at $20°C$ in the presence of acetylcholine at pH 11 formed 4-amino-4'-nitrobiphenyl.	19
Oxidation	Oxidation with chloramine-T was the basis for analysis. However, the colored product contained unoxidized benzidine. References were given to earlier oxidation procedures.	20
Oxidation Photo-decomposition	Oxidation by Co^{+3} in glacial HOAc occurred slowly. UV irradiation resulted in slow decomposition, the products varying with the solvent used. Products were not identified.	21

BENZIDINE (92-87-5)
(continued)

Degradation Technique	Remarks	Reference
Photo-decomposition	An analytical procedure was described. A dilute solution of benzidine in water lost only about 11% of the amine in 16 days under fluorescent lights at 25°C in glass bottles. The 2HCl salt decreased less than 2% under the same conditions.	22
Photo-decomposition Microbial	Irradiation in methanol at 254 nm gave a $T_{1/2}$ of about 2 hr. Laboratory model ecosystems were used for studying the bioaccumulation and degradation of benzidine by various organisms. About 80% was degraded by soil microbes in four weeks at 26.7°C.	23
Microbial	Oxidation by activated sludge was used for the treatment of wastewater. Included other aromatic amines.	24
Ozonation	Short periods of ozonation eliminated the need for metabolic activation of benzidine in the Ames mutagenesis assay. Further ozonation destroyed the mutagenicity when tested in the presence or absence of microsomal activation. No details.	25
Microbial	Acclimated aeration sludges completely oxidized continuous doses of 1 mg benzidine per liter. Less complete degradation occurred at higher levels. Concentrations less than 1 mg/ℓ are probably degraded by natural ecosystems.	26

Benzidine

1. Genin, V. A. Decontamination of industrial effluents containing benzidine. *Gig. Sanit.* **38**(3):105–107, 1973.
2. *Int. Agency Res. Cancer Monogr.* 1:80, Lyon, France, 1972.
3. Lurie, A. P. Benzidine and related diaminobiphenyls. In: *Kirk-Othmer: Encyclopedia of Chemical Technology, 2nd ed.* 3:408–420. John Wiley & Sons, New York, 1964.

4. Butt, L. T. and Strafford, N. Papilloma of the bladder in the chemical industry. Analytical methods for the determination of benzidine and β-naphthylamine, recommended by A. B. C. M. sub-committee. *J. Appl. Chem.* 6:525–539, 1956.

5. Iwanami, Y. The reaction of acetylenecarboxylic acid with amines. XVII. The addition of dialkyl acetylenedicarboxylates to several carcinogens. *Bull. Chem. Soc. Jpn.* 48:1657–1658, 1975.

6. Volodina, M. A. and Khryashchevskaya, O. M. Decomposition of benzidine, hydrazobenzene, and azobenzene in a high-frequency discharge in hydrogen in the presence of silver chloride. *Vestn Mosk. Univ. Khim.* 17:586–590, 1976.

7. *The Merck Index, 9th ed.*: entry #1083, Windholz, M., Buavari, S., Stroumtsos, L. Y., and Fertig, M. N. (Eds.). Merck and Co., Rahway, New Jersey, 1976.

8. Umbraziunaite, O. and Jasinskiene, E. Use of benzidine and its derivatives for determining iodides by a kinetic method. *Nauchn. Konf. Khim.-Anal. Pribalt. Resp. B SSR (Tezisy Dokl), 1st:* 204–206, 1974.

9. Barek, J. and Berka, A. Oxidation of benzidine, o,o'-tolidine and o,o'-dianisidine using a diphosphate complex of trivalent manganese and manganese (III) sulfate. *Collect. Czech. Chem. Commun.* 41:1334–1342, 1976.

10. Barek, J. and Berka, A. Oxidation of organic substances with compounds of trivalent manganese. VI. Oxidation of benzidine, o-tolidine and o-dianisidine with a diphosphate complex of trivalent manganese in buffer medium. *Collect. Czech. Chem. Commun.* 42:1949–1959, 1977.

11. Pshezhetskii, V. S. and Yaroslavov, A. A. Synthetic high-molecular-weight catalysts as functional analogs of peroxidase. *Bioorg. Khim.* 3:1117–1125, 1977.

12. Dolmanova, I. F., Zolotova, G. A., Shekhovtsova, T. N., and Peshkova, V. M. Mechanism of the catalytic action of chromium in oxidation reactions of benzidine derivatives by hydrogen peroxide. *Zh. Anal. Khim.* 27:1403–1407, 1972.

13. Genin, V. A. Decontamination of working clothes contaminated with benzidine and dianisidine. *Bezop. Tr. Prom.* (2):23, 1973.

14. Kalinina, V. E. Kinetics and mechanism of periodate oxidation reactions catalyzed by ruthenium compounds. *Kinet. Katal.* 12:100–106, 1971.

15. Kalinina, V. E. and Yatsimirskii, K. B. Catalytic properties of ruthenium (III) and (IV) compounds in reactions of oxidation by periodate. *Anal. Tekhnol. Blagorod. Metal:* 123–128, 1971.

16. Matrka, M., Pipalova, J., Sagner, Z., and Marhold, J. Semiquinone formation during the oxidation of benzidine, o-tolidine, and o-dianisidine. *Chem. Prum.* 21:14–18, 1971.

17. Dohnal, L. and Zyka, J. The oxidation of benzidine, o,o'-tolidine and o,o'-dianisidine with cobalt (III) perchlorate. *Microchem. J.* 20:221–226, 1975.

64   Degradation of Chemical Carcinogens

18. Berka, A., Korinkova, M., and Barek, J. The oxidation of benzidine, o,o'-tolidine and o,o'-dianisidine by manganese dioxide. *Microchem. J.* **21**: 38–44, 1976.
19. Aksnes, G. and Sandberg, K. On the oxidation of benzidine and o-dianisidine with hydrogen peroxide and acetylcholine in alkaline solution. *Acta Chem. Scand.* **11**:876–880, 1957.
20. Glassman, J. M. and Meigs, J. W. Benzidine (4,4'-diaminobiphenyl) and substituted benzidines. *Arch. Ind. Hyg. Occup. Med.* **4**:519–532, 1951.
21. Dohnal, L. and Zyka, J. A study of oxidation of benzidine, o,o'-tolidine, and o,o'-dianisidine. *Microchem. J.* **19**:63–70, 1974.
22. Bowman, M. C., King, J. R., and Holder, C. L. Benzidine and congeners: analytical chemical properties and trace analysis in five substrates. *Int. J. Environ. Anal. Chem.* **4**:205–223, 1976.
23. Lu, P.-Y., Metcalf, R. L., Plummer, N., and Mandel, D. The environmental fate of three carcinogens: benzo(a)pyrene, benzidine, and vinyl chloride evaluated in laboratory model ecosystems. *Arch. Environ. Contam. Toxicol.* **6**:129–142, 1977.
24. Baird, R., Carmona, L., and Jenkins, R. L. Behavior of benzidine and other aromatic amines in aerobic wastewater treatment. *J. Water Pollut. Control Fed.* **49**:1609–1615, 1977.
25. Caulfield, M. J. and Burleson, G. R. Inactivation of carcinogens by ozonation as monitored by the Ames mutagenesis assay. *Fed. Proc., Fed. Am. Soc. Exp. Biol.* **36**:1079, 1977.
26. Tabak, H. H. and Barth, E. F. Biodegradability of benzidine in aerobic suspended growth reactors. *J. Water Pollut. Control Fed.* **50**:552–558, 1978.

3,3'-DICHLOROBENZIDINE (91-94-1)

Degradation Technique	Remarks	Reference
Bromination	Introduction of Br into the 5 and 5' positions eliminated the carcinogenicity, presumably by preventing the production of carcinogenic metabolites.	1
Oxidation	Incomplete oxidation with chloramine-T was the basis for colorimetric analysis.	2
Photo-decomposition	UV irradiation in aqueous solution caused a rapid degradation to monochlorobenzidine, benzidine, and several unidentified, colored products, which were adsorbed to the walls of the photoreactor. The reaction was considerably slower in organic solvents.	3

3,3'-Dichlorobenzidine

1. Pliss, G. B. Effect of bromination on the carcinogenic properties of 3,3'-dichlorobenzidine. *Vopr. Onkol.* 21:110–112, 1975.
2. Glassman, J. M. and Meigs, J. W. Benzidine (4,4'-diaminobiphenyl) and substituted benzidines. *Arch. Ind. Hyg. Occup. Med.* 4:519–532, 1951.
3. Banerjee, S., Sikka, H. C., Gray, R., and Kelly, C. M. Photodegradation of 3,3'-dichlorobenzidine. *Environ. Sci. Technol.* 12:1425–1427, 1978.

3,3'-DIMETHOXYBENZIDINE (119-90-4)

Degradation Technique	Remarks	Reference
Oxidation	Oxidation by commercial horseradish peroxidase and H_2O_2 in phosphate buffer at 21°C was used in a study of anti-inflammatory drugs.	1
Oxidation	Oxidation by commercial horseradish peroxidase and H_2O_2 in phosphate buffer was used in a study of venom activities. The product was the quinone diimine.	2

3,3'-DIMETHOXYBENZIDINE (119-90-4)
(continued)

Degradation Technique	Remarks	Reference
Oxidation	A kinetic study of the oxidation by H_2O_2 in the presence of horseradish peroxidase at pH 3.7–9.0.	3
Oxidation	Iodide catalyzed the oxidation by H_2O_2.	4
Oxidation	Mn^{+3} was used for the oxidation, which produced the quinone diimine.	5
Oxidation	The mechanism of oxidation by Mn^{+3} was further studied.	6
Oxidation	A kinetic study of the oxidation by H_2O_2, catalyzed by Cr ions.	7
Oxidation	A kinetic study of the oxidation by periodate, catalyzed by Mn^{+2} ions.	8
Oxidation	Oxidation by H_2O_2 was catalyzed by several metal ions.	9
Oxidation	A kinetic study of the oxidation by periodate, catalyzed by Ru ions.	10
Oxidation	The effect of pH was included in this study of the oxidation by periodate, catalyzed by Ru ions.	11
Oxidation	A study of semiquinone formation during the oxidation with $Ce(SO_4)_2$ and Br_2 at pH 0–9.	12
Oxidation	Oxidation by $Co(ClCO_4)_3$ produced a red precipitate, which was not identified.	13
Oxidation	Hydrated MnO_2 produced a quantitative oxidation to the quinione diimine in dilute HCl at room temperature.	14
Oxidation	Oxidation by H_2O_2 at $20°C$ in the presence of acetylcholine at pH 11 led to the formation of three products, which were identified.	15
Oxidation	Incomplete oxidation with chloramine-T was the basis for colorimetric analysis.	16

3,3'-DIMETHOXYBENZIDINE (119-90-4)
(continued)

Degradation Technique	Remarks	Reference
Oxidation	Oxidation by H_2O_2 was catalyzed by Cr ions and further activated by certain organic compounds.	17
Oxidation	A solution of 2.5% NaOCl was recommended for decontaminating work clothes.	18
Oxidation Photo-decomposition	Oxidation by Co^{+3} in glacial HOAc occurred slowly. UV irradiation resulted in slow decomposition, the products varying with the solvent used. Products were not identified.	19
Photo-decomposition	A dilute aqueous solution of the free amine lost about 64% in 16 days under fluorescent lights at 25°C in glass bottles. The 2HCl salt lost only about 9% under the same conditions.	20
Demethylation	Treatment with 50% H_2SO_4 at 180°C for 10 hr under N_2 gave dihydroxybenzidine.	21
Demethylation	Treatment with concentrated HCl in an autoclave at 150°C for 8 hr gave about 61% dihydroxybenzidine.	22
	First aid and disposal of spills were described.	23

3,3'-Dimethoxybenzidine

1. Saeed, S. A. and Warren, B. T. On the mode of action and biochemical properties of anti-inflammatory drugs. I. *Biochem. Pharmacol.* 22:1965–1969, 1973.
2. Tu, A. T. and Passey, R. B. Effect of *Naja naja atra* venom on cytochrome C oxidase, *L*-ascorbic acid oxidase, peroxidase, and catalase. *Toxicon.* 3: 25–31, 1965.
3. Lebedeva, O. V., Ugarova, N. N., and Berezin, I. V. Kinetic study of *o*-dianisidine oxidation by hydrogen peroxide in the presence of horseradish peroxidase. *Biokhimiya* 42:1372–1379, 1977.

 4. Umbraziunaite, O. and Jasinskiene, E. Use of benzidine and its derivatives for determining iodides by a kinetic method. *Nauchn. Konf. Khim.-Anal. Pribalt. Resp. B SSR (Tezisy Dokl), 1st:* 204-206, 1974.
 5. Barek, J. and Berka, A. Oxidation of benzidine, *o,o'*-tolidine and *o,o'*-dianisidine using a diphosphate complex of trivalent manganese and manganese (III) sulfate. *Collect. Czech. Chem. Commun.* 41:1334-1342, 1976.
 6. Barek, J. and Berka, A. Oxidation of organic substances with compounds of trivalent manganese. VI. Oxidation of benzidine, *o*-tolidine and *o*-dianisidine with a diphosphate complex of trivalent manganese in buffer medium. *Collect. Czech. Chem. Commun.* 42:1949-1959, 1977.
 7. Dolmanova, I. F., Zolotova, G. A., Shekhovtsova, T. N., and Peshkova, V. M. Mechanism of the catalytic action of chromium in oxidation reactions of benzidine derivatives by hydrogen peroxide. *Zh. Anal. Khim.* 27:1403-1407, 1972.
 8. Dolmanova, I. F., Yatsimirskaya, N. T., and Peshkova, V. M. Mechanism of the catalytic action of manganese (II) in the oxidation of *o*-dianisidine by periodate. *Kinet. Katal.* 13:678-684, 1972.
 9. Abe, S., Takahashi, K., and Matsuo, T. Manganese (II) catalyzed oxidation of aromatic amines by hydrogen peroxide and its application to the chelatometric determination of manganese. *Nippon Kagaku Kaishi:* 963-967, 1973.
10. Kalinina, V. E. Kinetics and mechanism of periodate oxidation reactions catalyzed by ruthenium compounds. *Kinet. Katal.* 12:100-106, 1971.
11. Kalinina, V. E. and Yatsimirskii, K. B. Catalytic properties of ruthenium (III) and (IV) compounds in reactions of oxidation by periodate. *Anal. Tekhnol. Blagorod. Metal:* 123-128, 1971.
12. Matrka, M., Pipalova, J., Sagner, Z., and Marhold, J. Semiquinone formation during the oxidation of benzidine, *o*-tolidine, and *o*-dianisidine. *Chem. Prum.* 21:14-18, 1971.
13. Dohnal, L. and Zyka, J. The oxidation of benzidine, *o,o'*-tolidine and *o,o'*-dianisidine with cobalt (III) perchlorate. *Microchem. J.* 20:221-226, 1975.
14. Berka, A., Korinkova, M., and Barek, J. The oxidation of benzidine, *o,o'*-tolidine and *o,o'*-dianisidine by manganese dioxide. *Microchem. J.* 21:38-44, 1976.
15. Aksnes, G. and Sandberg, K. On the oxidation of benzidine and *o*-dianisidine with hydrogen peroxide and acetylcholine in alkaline solution. *Acta Chem. Scand.* 11:876-880, 1957.
16. Glassman, J. M. and Meigs, J. W. Benzidine (4,4'-diaminobiphenyl) and substituted benzidines. *Arch. Ind. Hyg. Occup. Med.* 4:519-532, 1951.
17. Dolmanova, I. F. and Shekhovtsova, T. N. Mechanism of activator action in the reaction between *o*-dianisidine and hydrogen peroxide catalyzed by chromium. *Zh. Anal. Khim.* 32:1154-1158, 1977.

18. Genin, V. A. Decontamination of working clothes contaminated with benzidine and dianisidine. *Bezop. Tr. Prom.* (2):23, 1973.
19. Dohnal, L. and Zyka, J. A study of oxidation of benzidine, *o,o'*-tolidine, and *o,o'*-dianisidine. *Microchem. J.* **19**:63–70, 1974.
20. Bowman, M. C., King, J. R., and Holder, C. L. Benzidine and congeners: analytical chemical properties and trace analysis in five substrates. *Int. J. Environ. Anal. Chem.* **4**:205–223, 1976.
21. Hagiwara, Y., Kurihara, M., Kobayashi, A., and Yoda, N. Aromatic hydroxy amines. *Japanese Patent #74-33,186,* Sept. 5, 1974.
22. Hagiwara, Y., Kurihara, M., Kobayashi, A., and Yoda, N. Aromatic hydroxy amines. *Japanese Patent #74-33,187,* Sept. 5, 1974.
23. *Hazards in the Chemical Laboratory, 2nd ed.:* 235, Muir, G. D. (Ed.), The Chemical Society, London, 1977.

3,3'-DIMETHYLBENZIDINE (119-93-7)

Degradation Technique	Remarks	Reference
Oxidation	Iodide catalyzed the oxidation by H_2O_2.	1
Oxidation	Mn^{+3} was used for the oxidation, which produced the quinone diimine.	2
Oxidation	A kinetic study of the oxidation by H_2O_2, catalyzed by Cr ions.	3
Oxidation	Oxidation by H_2O_2 was catalyzed by several metal ions.	4
Oxidation	A kinetic study of the oxidation by periodate, catalyzed by Ru ions.	5
Oxidation	A study of semiquinone formation during the oxidation with $Ce(SO_4)_2$ and Br_2 at pH 0–9.	6
Oxidation	$Co(ClO_4)_3$ produced the quinone diimine without any semiquinone.	7
Oxidation	Hydrated MnO_2 produced a quantitative oxidation to the quinone diimine in dilute HCl at room temperature.	8
Oxidation	Incomplete oxidation with chloramine-T was the basis for colorimetric analysis.	9

3,3'-DIMETHYLBENZIDINE (119-93-7)
(continued)

Degradation Technique	Remarks	Reference
Oxidation Photo-decomposition	Oxidation by Co^{+3} in glacial HOAc occurred slowly. UV irradiation resulted in slow de-composition, the products varying with the solvent used. Products were not identified.	10
Photo-decomposition	A dilute aqueous solution of the free amine or its 2HCl salt lost about 9% of the compound in 16 days under fluorescent lights at 25°C in glass bottles.	11
Oxidation Tetrazotization Acetylation	No details.	12
	First aid and handling of spills were described.	13

3,3'-Dimethylbenzidine

1. Umbraziunaite, O. and Jasinskiene, E. Use of benzidine and its derivatives for determining iodides by a kinetic method. *Nauchn. Konf. Khim.-Anal. Pribalt. Resp. B SSR (Tezisky Dokl), 1st:* 204–206, 1974.
2. Barek, J. and Berka, A. Oxidation of benzidine, o,o'-tolidine and o,o'-dianisidine using a diphosphate complex of trivalent manganese and manganese (III) sulfate. *Collect, Czech. Chem. Commun.* 41:1334–1342, 1976.
3. Dolmanova, I. F., Zolotova, G. A., Shekovtsova, T. N., and Peshkova, V. M. Mechanism of the catalytic action of chromium in oxidation reactions of benzidine derivatives by hydrogen peroxide. *Zh. Anal. Khim.* 27:1403–1407, 1972.
4. Abe, S., Takahashi, K., and Matsuo, T. Manganese (II) catalyzed oxidation of aromatic amines by hydrogen peroxide and its application to the chelatometric determination of manganese. *Nippon Kagaku Kaishi:* 963–967, 1973.
5. Kalinina, V. E. Kinetics and mechanism of periodate oxidation reactions catalyzed by ruthenium compounds. *Kinet. Katal.* 12:100–106, 1971.
6. Matrka, M., Pipalova, J., Sagner, Z., and Marhold, J. Semiquinone formation during the oxidation of benzidine, o-tolidine, and o-dianisidine. *Chem. Prum.* 21:14–18, 1971.
7. Dohnal, L. and Zyka, J. The oxidation of benzidine, o,o'-tolidine and o,o'-dianisidine with cobalt (III) perchlorate. *Microchem. J.* 20:221–226, 1975.

8. Berka, A., Korinkova, M., and Barek, J. The oxidation of benzidine, o,o'-tolidine and o,o'-dianisidine by manganese dioxide. *Microchem. J.* 21:38–44, 1976.
9. Glassman, J. M. and Meigs, J. W. Benzidine (4,4'-diaminobiphenyl) and substituted benzidines. *Arch. Ind. Hyg. Occup. Med.* 4:519–532, 1951.
10. Dohnal, L. and Zyka, J. A study of oxidation of benzidine, o,o'-tolidine, and o,o'-dianisidine. *Microchem. J.* 19:63–70, 1974.
11. Bowman, M. C., King, J. R., and Holder, C. L. Benzidine and congeners: analytical chemical properties and trace analysis in five substrates. *Int. J. Environ, Anal. Chem.* 4:205–223, 1976.
12. *Int. Agency Res. Cancer Monogr.* 1:87, Lyon, France, 1972.
13. *Hazards in the Chemical Laboratory, 2nd ed.:* 409, Muir, G. D. (Ed.). The Chemical Society, London, 1977.

4,4'-METHYLENE BIS(2-CHLOROANILINE) (101-14-4)

Degradation Technique	Remarks	Reference
Reaction with sulfamic acid	1% Sulfamic acid in 0.5% surfactant was used for decontaminating equipment and work areas. Safety of the amine sulfamate product was not assured.	1

4,4'-Methylene bis(2-chloroaniline)

1. Schmitt, C. R. and Cagle, G. W. Sulfamic acid cleaning solution for 4,4'-methylene-bis-orthochloroaniline (MOCA). *J. Am. Ind. Hyg. Assoc.* 36:181–186, 1975.

1-NAPHTHYLAMINE (134-32-7)
2-NAPHTHYLAMINE (91-59-8)

Degradation Technique	Remarks	Reference
Oxidation	Oxidation of 2-naphthylamine by $K_2S_2O_8$ gave 2-NH_2-1-naphthyl KSO_4 at pH 7.5.	1
Oxidation	Primary aromatic amines were oxidized by nitrosodisulfonate. The toxicity of the reagent and products was not discussed.	2

1-NAPHTHYLAMINE (134–32–7)
2-NAPHTHYLAMINE (91–59–8)
(continued)

Degradation Technique	Remarks	Reference
Oxidation	2-Naphthylamine was oxidized by peroxidase or by Fe^{+2} and H_2O_2. Some products were identified.	3
Oxidation	A review with 142 references. The detailed mechanism of the oxidation of 1-naphthylamine with $Ce(SO_4)_2$ was given.	4
Oxidation	The stoichiometry and a reaction scheme were given for the oxidation of 1-naphthylamine with $Ce(SO_4)_2$.	5
Oxidation	Oxidation of 1-naphthylamine by BrO^- was catalyzed by V and Mo at pH 1.85.	6
Oxidation	A number of products were identified after the oxidation of 2-naphthylamine by benzoyl peroxide at $80°C$. References to other oxidation studies were cited.	7
Oxidation	Oxidation of 1-naphthylamine by percapric acid was catalyzed by Ni^{+2} at pH 12.7.	8
Oxidation	1-Naphthylamine was titrated in acid isopropanol using Cu electrodes.	9
Photo-decomposition	Both isomers are sensitive to light. No details.	10
Photo-decomposition	An orange-brown oxidation product formed when 2-naphthylamine was exposed to light in the presence of air. It differed from the three major oxidation products previously reported.	11
Photo-decomposition	Irradiation of a methanolic solution of 2-naphthylamine at 254 nm produced a red compound (2-amino-1,4-naphthoquinone-N^4, 2-naphthylimine), which may be responsible for the carcinogenic activity of 2-naphthylamine.	12
Chemical	Decomposition products of both isomers were prepared and their carcinogenicities were tested in several animal species.	13

1-NAPHTHYLAMINE (134-32-7)
2-NAPHTHYLAMINE (91-59-8)
(continued)

Degradation Technique	Remarks	Reference
Chemical	Standard reactions of primary aromatic amines were described and used as bases for analyses: oxidation with NaOCl; diazotization and coupling with 2,3-hydroxynaphthoic acid or R-salt.	14
Deamination	Naphthylamines were diazotized, complexed with $HgBr_2$, and decomposed to the corresponding naphthalenes.	15
Reaction with p-diazobenzenesulfonic acid	1-Naphthylamine reacted to form the azo dye. Method for analysis of selenium.	16
Reaction with dialkyl acetylenedicarboxylates	The addition of dialkyl acetylenedicarboxylates to carcinogenic amines was described. 1-Naphthylamine reacted almost quantitatively. The product was to be tested for carcinogenicity.	17
Reaction with allyl bromide	The rate constants were determined for 2-naphthylamine at 70°C and 80°C.	18
	First aid and handling of spills of 1-naphthylamine are described.	19

1-Naphthylamine and 2-Naphthylamine

1. Manson, D. Isolation of 2-amino-1-naphthyl hydrogen sulphate with cetylpyridinium bromide from metabolic and chemical oxidations of 2-naphthylamine. *Biochem. J.* 119:541-546, 1970.
2. Tueber, H.-J. and Jellinek, G. Reactions with nitrosodisulfonate. VII. Oxidation of primary aromatic amines. *Chem. Ber.* 87:1841-1848, 1954.
3. Saunders, B. C. and Wodak, J. Studies in peroxidase action. XIII. The oxidation of 2-naphthylamine. *Tetrahedron* 22:505-508, 1966.
4. Velich, V. Oxidation mechanism of 1-naphthylamine with cerium (IV) sulfate in aqueous solutions of sulfuric and hydrochloric acids. *Sb. Ved. Pr. Vys. Sk. Chemickotechnol Pardubice* 18:173-229, 1968.

5. Tockstein, A., Velich, V., and Komers, K. Cerimetric oxidation of 1-naphthylamine and 8-aminonaphthalene-1-sulfonic acid in aqueous acid solution. I. Reaction mechanism. *Collect. Czech. Chem. Commun.* 34:3017–3032, 1969.

6. Kuz'mina, A. E., Kolosov, I. V., and Andreeva, Z. F. Optimum conditions for determining trace amounts of molybdenum and vanadium by a kinetic method. *Izv. Timiryazev Sel'skokhoz Akad.:* 228–230, 1970.

7. Orr, S. F. D., Sims, P., and Manson, D. The oxidation of 2-naphthylamine with benzoyl peroxide. *J. Chem. Soc.:* 1337–1344, 1956.

8. Skorobogatyi, Ya. P., Zinchuk, V. K., and Markovskaya, R. F. Use of the oxidation of α-naphthylamine by percapric acid for kinetic determination of trace amounts of nickel. In: *Org. Reagenty Anal. Khim. Tezisy Dokl. Vses. Konf., 4th* 2:71–72, 1976.

9. Shvyrkova, L. A. and Burakova, T. P. Biamperometric titration of amines. *Tr. Mosk. Khim.-Tekhnol. Inst.* 81:100–101, 1974.

10. *The Merck Index 9th ed.:* entries #6225 and 6226, Windholz, M., Buavari, S., Stroumtsos, L. Y., and Fertig, M. N. (Eds.). Merck and Co., Rahway, New Jersey, 1976.

11; Osteen, A. F. *The Photosensitizing Action of 2-Naphthylamine on Escherichia coli K-12.* U.S. NTIS PB Rep. 242340, pp. 35–41, Springfield, Virginia, 1973.

12. Brill, E. and Radomski, J. L. 2-Amino-1,4-naphthoquinone-N[4], 2-naphthylimine. A photo-oxidation product of 2-aminonaphthalene. *Experientia* 21:368–369, 1965.

13. Radomski, J. L., Brill, E., Deichmann, W. B., and Glass, E. M. Carcinogenicity testing of N-hydroxy and other oxidation and decomposition products of 1- and 2-naphthylamine. *Cancer Res.* 31:1461–1467, 1971.

14. Butt, L. T. and Strafford, N. Papilloma of the bladder in the chemical industry. Analytical methods for the determination of benzidine and β-naphthylamine, recommended by A. B. C. M. sub-committee. *J. Appl. Chem.* 6:525–539, 1956.

15. Newman, M. S. and Hung, W. M. A new method for deamination of naphthylamines. *J. Org. Chem.* 39:1317, 1974.

16. Kawashima, T., Nakano, S., and Tanaka, M. Catalytic determination of submicrogram amounts of selenium (IV) by means of the oxidative coupling reaction of phenylhydrazine-*p*-sulfonic acid with 1-naphthylamine. *Anal. Chim. Acta* 49:443–447, 1970.

17. Iwanami, Y. The reaction of acetylenecarboxylic acid with amines. XVII. The addition of dialkyl acetylenedicarboxylates to several carcinogens. *Bull. Chem. Soc. Jpn.* 48:1657–1658, 1975.

18. Panigrahi, G. P. and Sinha, T. K. Structure-reactivity correlation in the reaction of aliphatic and aromatic amines with allyl bromide and allyl chloride. *Indian J. Chem.* **15B**:561–562, 1977.
19. *Hazards in the Chemical Laboratory, 2nd ed.:* 325, Muir, G. D. (Ed.). The Chemical Society, London, 1977.

m-TOLUENEDIAMINE (95-80-7)

Degradation Technique	Remarks	Reference
Hydrolysis	Methylresorcinols were formed by the hydrolysis of toluenediamines with aqueous NH_4HSO_4 at elevated temperature.	1
Microbial	*m*-Toluenediamine was included in a group of organic compounds relatively easily decomposed by activated sludge in the treatment of waste-water.	2
Oxidation	Electrolytic oxidation occurred in acid isopropanol with Cu electrodes.	3
Reaction with HCHO and oxidation	Reaction with HCHO at 60°C for 1 hr, followed by oxidation with NaOCl, was used for degradation in aqueous solutions.	4
Reaction with aldehydes	Reaction with benzaldehyde at 50°C in aqueous HCl gave the addition product.	5
Acetylation	Conditions for acetylation were listed and physicochemical properties of the products were described. Toxicities of the products were not given.	6

m-Toluenediamine

1. Greco, N. P. Hydrolysis of toluene diamines to produce methyl resorcinols. U.S. Patent #3,933,925, Jan. 20, 1976.
2. Matsui, S., Murakami, T., Sasaki, T., Hirose, Y., and Iguma, Y. Activated sludge degradability of organic substances in the waste water of the Kashima Petroleum and Petrochemical Industrial Complex in Japan. *Prog. Water Technol.* 7:645–659, 1975.
3. Shvyrkova, L. A. and Burakova, T. P. Biamperometric titration of amines. *Tr. Mosk. Khim.-Tekhnol. Inst.* 81:100–101, 1974.
4. Oda, N., Horie, Y., Idohara, M., Namioka, T., and Yahata, A. Treatment of amine-containing waste water or solution. *Japanese Patent #76-28,358,* March 10, 1976.
5. Ziemek, P. Condensation products of hydrophobic aldehydes with aromatic amines. *German Patent #2,308,724,* Sept. 12, 1974.
6. Glinsukon, T., Weisburger, E. K., Benjamin, T., and Roller, P. P. Preparation and spectra of some acetyl derivatives of 2,4-toluenediamine. *J. Chem. Eng. Data* 20:207–209, 1975.

ARYL HALIDES

POLYCHLORINATED BIPHENYLS
(1336-36-3: UNSPECIFIED STRUCTURE)

Degradation Technique	Remarks	Reference
Chemical Thermal	Aroclors are not hydrolyzed by water; resist alkalies, acids, and other corrosive chemicals; and are resistant to long periods of heating.	1
Chemical Thermal Oxidation	PCB's are not hydrolyzed by water; resist heat, alkali, acid, etc. Burning created more toxic products. Included chronic toxicity studies.	2
Physical Chemical Biodegradation	A definitive text on the chemistry of PCB's.	3
Biodegradation Oxidation	No degradation was produced by algae or by conventional oxidation treatments of water. Large amounts of activated C removed most of the PCB's.	4
	A variety of adsorbents was studied for removing Aroclor 1242 and 1254 from wastewater. PVC was very effective. Studies were to be made for the regeneration of the PVC and degradation of the PCB's.	5
	A water treatment system was described for the elimination of pesticides and PCB's by chlorination, flocculation, filtration, and adsorption.	6
Physical Chemical	A review of the treatment and disposal of PCB's by various dechlorination procedures.	7
Physical Chemical	Decomposition was effected by irradiation or heating $\pm$ O_2 $\pm$ organic peracids. UV irradiation in alkaline isopropanol for 15 min at 30°C under N_2 completely decomposed PCB.	8
Physical Chemical Microbial	Photolytic, radiolytic, thermal, hydrolytic, and microbial procedures were discussed.	9

POLYCHLORINATED BIPHENYLS
(1336-36-3: UNSPECIFIED STRUCTURE)
(continued)

Degradation Technique	Remarks	Reference
Ionizing radiation	Alkali catalyzed the dechlorination of PCB's by ^{60}Co irradiation.	10
Ionizing radiation	A review of the radiolytic dechlorination of PCB's. The use of other energy sources was discussed.	11
Ionizing radiation	Solutions of PCB's were exposed to ^{60}Co irradiation. Dechlorination was greater than that produced by photolysis. Organic chloride pesticides were included in the study.	12
Ionizing radiation	Ten Mrad gamma radiation (^{60}Co) destroyed 92% of the PCB in an aqueous solution containing 100 ppb. Acute toxicity for shrimps disappeared after treatment.	13
Photo-decomposition	Cl atoms were removed when a hexachlorobiphenyl in hexane was irradiated with 310 nm light for 100 min.	14
Photo-decomposition	UV degradation was catalyzed by diethylamine. Complete degradation occurred during 100 min irradiation, depending on the concentration of PCB's.	15
Photo-decomposition	Sun-drying fish in the presence of $NaNO_2$ slightly hastened the dechlorination of contaminating PCB's by a few hours.	16
Photo-decomposition	Irradiation with UV at 300 nm caused dechlorination. Products were studied.	17
Photo-decomposition	Dechlorination, polymerization, and oxidation occurred. Products were studied.	18
Photo-decomposition	A review chapter. Photochemical degradation of PCB's can form less toxic and more toxic products.	19
Photo-decomposition	Irradiation with UV light was used to form degradation products for GLC analysis of PCB's.	20

POLYCHLORINATED BIPHENYLS
(1336-36-3: UNSPECIFIED STRUCTURE)
(continued)

Degradation Technique	Remarks	Reference
Photo-decomposition	Partial dechlorination of a dichloro- and a tetrachlorobiphenyl occurred during prolonged irriadation in hexane at about 310 nm.	21
Photo-decomposition	PCB's were destroyed when irradiated by 365 nm UV light in the presence of a suspension of TiO_2. Cl^{-1} was liberated during the degradation.	22
Photo-decomposition	UV irradiation (300 nm) dechlorinated tetra-chlorobiphenyls. Cl atoms in *para* positions were less readily attacked than those in the *ortho* or *meta* isomers.	23
Photo-decomposition	PCB's were dechlorinated by UV irradiation in alkaline isopropanol solution.	24
Photo-decomposition	The mechanism and safety of PCB dechlorination by UV light were discussed.	25
Photo-decomposition	UV irradiation of PCB's was studied in solutions, solid, and gas phases. Dechlorination, isomerization, and biphenyl splitting occurred. Higher molecular weight products also formed by the introduction of more Cl atoms, as well as O and N.	26
Photo-decomposition	Ten GLC peaks of Aroclor 1254 were followed during irradiation with UV or sunlight. All peaks disappeared in 30 min with UV treatment of a solution in hexane. Degradation was less effective in water or benzene and with sunlight. The possibility of forming products more toxic than the parent compounds was mentioned.	27
Photo-decomposition	2,2'-Dichlorobiphenyl reacted at 40-50°C with the intermediates generated from N_2O to form dichlorohydroxybiphenyl and chloronitrobiphenylol.	28

POLYCHLORINATED BIPHENYLS
(1336-36-3: UNSPECIFIED STRUCTURE)
(continued)

Degradation Technique	Remarks	Reference
Photo-decomposition	Slow dechlorination of low molecular weight PCB's occurred when aqueous suspensions were exposed to a UV lamp or sunlight.	29
Photo-decomposition Microbial	A review of the degradation of ten pesticides in aquatic systems. PCB's were not readily degraded. No details.	30
Photo-decomposition Oxidation	A history of the discovery of the contamination of the environment by PCB's with references to their stability and degradation by UV and incineration.	31
Oxidation	An incineration plant was described for the degradation of chemical wastes, including PCB's, at 1,000–1,200°C. Flue gases were purified by scrubbers.	32
Oxidation	At 950°C, under specified conditions, PCB's were destroyed rapidly, yielding simple inorganic substances.	33
Oxidation	Efficient destruction of Aroclor 1254 occurred during normal operation of a multiple hearth furnace (625°C afterburner). No PCB was found in the scrubber effluent or ash, and less than 6% escaped in the flue gas.	34
Oxidation	PCB's and other chlorinated organic compounds were completely decomposed by heating with steam in a C-filled reactor at 800°C.	35
Oxidation	Practically 100% destruction of PCB's occurred during commercial incineration of electrical capacitors.	36
Oxidation	Trichlorobiphenyl was mostly converted into HCl and C by repeatedly heating at 400°C in a mixture of molten salts through which air was passed.	37

POLYCHLORINATED BIPHENYLS
(1336-36-3: UNSPECIFIED STRUCTURE)
(continued)

Degradation Technique	Remarks	Reference
Oxidation	Hydroxyl and quinone derivatives were formed when PCB's were oxidized at a Pt electrode.	38
Oxidation	A study was made of the electrochemical oxidation of PCB's in acetonitrile.	39
Oxidation	Refluxing PCB's with HNO_3 (d.1.4) for 100 hr produced benzoic acid derivatives.	40
Microbial	Using an aerated sludge system, a high percentage of added PCB was removed from wastewater. However, it was not believed to be degraded, but rather dissolved in fats in the sludge, adsorbed on particulate matter, or ingested by microbial cells.	41
Microbial	The degradation rate of PCB's by activated sludge cultures decreased with increase in chlorine content. Mono- and dichloro biphenyls were readily degraded.	42
Microbial	Aroclor 1221 was completely degraded in one month at $20°C$ by bacteria isolated from lake water. The rate of degradation decreased with increased Cl content. The position of Cl also affected the degradation rate.	43
Microbial	Bacteria isolated from lake water slowly degraded Aroclor 1242 to give aliphatic and aromatic hydrocarbons as the major products.	44
Microbial	A pure culture of *Achromobacter*, isolated from sewage, was able to degrade various PCB's.	45
Microbial	Two species of *Achromobacter* were isolated from sewage. Washed cell suspensions degraded PCB's without dechlorination.	46
Microbial	An *Alcaligenes* species isolated from lake sediment degraded highly chlorinated PCB's less rapidly than those with less Cl. PCB's with no Cl in one ring were degraded faster than those in which this element occurred in both rings.	47

POLYCHLORINATED BIPHENYLS
(1336-36-3: UNSPECIFIED STRUCTURE)
(continued)

Degradation Technique	Remarks	Reference
Microbial	PCB's with up to six Cl atoms were degraded by microorganisms, but lower Cl content favored degradation. Some PCB's were more readily degraded as mixtures than when pure.	48
Microbial	Unsubstituted biphenyl was hydroxylated and cleaved by bacteria. A similar degradation of PCB's was postulated. No details.	49
Microbial	A study of the metabolism of 4-chlorobiphenyl by soil bacteria to form phenolic derivatives.	50
Microbial	A mixed culture of soil bacteria grown on benzene as sole C-source was incubated with PCB's for up to six weeks at 28–30°C. Chlorobenzoic acid derivatives accumulated.	51
Microbial	A *Pseudomonas* species, isolated from the Chesapeake Bay, degraded pure isomers and mixtures of PCB's. Up to 84% of Aroclor 1254 was degraded in 60 days.	52
Microbial	Aroclor 1254 was not degraded after nine weeks in moist soil at 25°C. Soil microflora appeared unable to degrade PCB's.	53
Microbial	2,2'-Dichlorobiphenyl was not degraded by any microorganisms or soil samples tested under several conditions of incubation at 25°C.	54
Reaction with Cl$_2$	PCB's and other organic compounds were reacted with Cl$_2$ in a pressure bomb. The reactions can be explosive.	55
Reaction with alkali	An alkaline decomposition method was used for determining PCB's in soil.	56
Reduction	Products identified after the electrolytic reductive dechlorination of 19 PCB's have 1–5 Cl atoms, all on one benzene ring.	57

POLYCHLORINATED BIPHENYLS
(1336-36-3: UNSPECIFIED STRUCTURE)
(continued)

Degradation Technique	Remarks	Reference
Reduction	Reductive dechlorination by H_2 occurred at less than $150°C$ in the presence of a Ni catalyst. Other chlorinated compounds were included.	58
Microwave discharge	Atomic O and free electrons in a reduced pressure plasma resulted in practically complete degradation and oxidation of PCB's to Cl_2, HCl, CO_2, CO, and water under the most favorable conditions for reaction.	59
Microbial	A detailed study was made of the effect of Cl content and position on the degradation of 31 PCB isomers by an *Alcaligenes* sp. and an *Acinetobacter* sp. Degradations were compared after incubating for 1 hr at pH 7.5 with bacteria previously grown with biphenyl or 4-Cl-biphenyl as sole C-sources. Degradation decreased as Cl content increased; monochlorobiphenyls were rapidly degraded with no parent compound remaining.	60
Oxidation	A study was made of PCB emissions from incinerators and from plants in which electrical equipment was filled. A 12-hearth incinerator destroyed 95–98.4% of the PCB's in sewage sludge, although the maximum temperature was only $870°C$. The efficiency was attributed to catalysis by metallic components in the sludge.	61
Oxidation	C_6Cl_6 was formed during the incineration of PCB's, more being produced at high temperatures (e.g., $1000°C$). C_6Cl_6 was partially degraded at $950°C$.	62

PCB: polychlorinated biphenyl   PVC: polyvinyl chloride

Polychlorinated Biphenyls

1. Willett, L. B. and Hess, J. F. Jr. Polychlorinated biphenyl residues in silos in the United States. In: *Residue Reviews* 55:135-147, Gunther, F. A. and Gunther, J. D. (Eds.). Springer-Verlag, New York, 1975.

2. Mauro, A. PCBs (polychlorobiphenyls) and the environment. *Ind. Aliment.* (*Pinerolo, Italy*) 13(11):97-100, 1973.

3. Hutzinger, O., Safe, S., and Zitko, V. *The Chemistry of PCB's.* CRC Press, Cleveland, Ohio, 1974.

4. Bauer, U. Polychlorinated biphenyls and water. *Gas-Wasserfach Wasser-Abwasser* 113(2):58-63, 1972.

5. Lawrence, J. and Tosine, H. M. Adsorption of polychlorinated biphenyls from aqueous solutions and sewage. *Environ. Sci. Technol.* 10:381-383, 1976.

6. Bauer, U. and Pfleger, R. Elimination of some pesticides and Clophen A 30 during water purification by chlorination, flocculation and filtration over activated carbon. *Gas-Wasserfach Wasser-Abwasser* 116:555-559, 1975.

7. Imanura, M. Treatment of polychlorinated biphenyls. *Kagaku* 28:581-586, 1973.

8. Shinozaki, Y., Sawai, T., Sawai, T., Yamanaka, S., Anda, K., Nishiwaki, T., and Ninomiya, A. Decomposition of polychlorinated biphenyls. *Japanese Patent #74-109,351,* 7 pp., Oct. 17, 1974.

9. Shinozaki, Y. Polychlorinated biphenyl, its properties and reactions. *Kagaku No Jikken* 24:1183-1194, 1973.

10. Sawai, T. Degradation of polychlorinated biphenyls (PCB) using radio-isotopes. *Genshiryoku Kogyo* 19(12):43-47, 1972.

11. Sawai, T. Decomposition of polychlorinated biphenyl by using radioiso-topes. *Genshiryoku Kogyo* 19(10):29-32, 1973.

12. Vollner, L. and Korte, F. Radiolysis of chloro-pesticides. II. Gamma radia-tion in hexane, acetone, and acetone/water. *Chemosphere* 3:275-280, 1974.

13. Sunada, T. Irradiation treatment of PCB in water. *Atoms in Japan* 6:7-9, 1972.

14. Safe, S. and Hutzinger, O. Polychlorinated biphenyls: photolysis of 2,4,6, 2',4',6'-hexachlorobiphenyl. *Nature* 232:641-642, 1971.

15. Lewis, R. G., Hanisch, R. C., MacLeod, K. E., and Sovocool, G. W. Photo-chemical confirmation of mirex in the presence of polychlorinated bi-phenyls. *J. Agric. Food Chem.* 24:1030-1035, 1976.

16. Khan, M. A., Novak, A. F., and Rao, R. M. Reduction of polychlorinated biphenyls in shrimp by physical and chemical methods. *J. Food Sci.* 41: 262-267, 1976.

17. Ruzo, L. O., Safe, S., and Zabik, M. J. Photodecomposition of unsym-metrical polychlorobiphenyls. *J. Agric. Food Chem.* 23:594-595, 1975.

18. Hutzinger, O., Safe, S., and Zitko, V. Photochemical degradation of chlorobiphenyls (PCBs). *Environ. Health Perspect.* 1:15–20, 1972.

19. Safe, S., Bunce, N. J., Chittim, B., Hutzinger, O., and Ruzo, L. O. Photodecomposition of halogenated aromatic compounds. In: *Identification and Analysis of Organic Pollutants in Water:* 35–47, Keith, L. H. (Ed.). Ann Arbor Science Publishers, Ann Arbor, Michigan, 1976.

20. Hannan, E. J., Bills, D. D., and Herring, J. L. Analysis of polychlorinated biphenyls by gas chromatography and ultraviolet irradiation. *J. Agric. Food Chem.* 21:87–90, 1973.

21. Ruzo, L. O., Zabik, M. J., and Schuetz, R. D. Polychlorinated biphenyls: photolysis of 3,4,3',4'-tetrachlorobiphenyl and 4,4'-dichlorobiphenyl in solution. *Bull. Environ. Contam. Toxicol.* 8:217–218, 1972.

22. Carey, J. H., Lawrence, J., and Tosine, H. M. Photodechlorination of PCB's in the presence of titanium dioxide in aqueous suspensions. *Bull. Environ. Contam. Toxicol.* 16:697–701, 1976.

23. Ruzo, L. O., Zabik, M. J., and Schuetz, R. D. Photochemistry of bioactive compounds. Photochemical processes of polychlorinated biphenyls. *J. Am. Chem. Soc.* 96:3809–3813, 1974.

24. Nishiwaki, T., Usui, M., Tsuda, M., and Anda, K. Dechlorination of polychlorinated biphenyl by UV-irradiation: effects of sodium chloride deposition on the lamp wall on the decomposition yield of PCB. *Tokyo-Torsitsu Kogyo Gijutsu Senta Kenkyu Hokoku* 5:91–96, 1975.

25. Sawai, T. Decomposition of PCB by chain dechlorination reaction. *Gendai Kagaku* 64:22–27, 1976.

26. Hustert, K. and Korte, F. Ecological chemistry. LXXVIII. Reactions of polychlorinated biphenyls during UV-irradiation. *Chemosphere* 3:153–156, 1974.

27. Herring, J. L., Hannan, E. J., and Bills, D. D. UV-irradiation of Aroclor 1254. *Bull. Environ. Contam. Toxicol.* 8:153–157, 1972.

28. Saravanja-Bozanic, V., Gäb, S., Hustert, K., and Korte, F. Ecological chemistry 133. Reactions of aldrin, chlordene and 2,2'-dichlorbiphenyl with O(^{3}P). *Chemosphere* 6:21–26, 1977.

29. Crosby, D. G. and Moilanen, K. W. Photodecomposition of chlorinated biphenyls II. Rate studies. *Bull. Environ. Contam. Toxicol.* 13:249–256, 377, 1973.

30. Paris, D. F. and Lewis, D. L. Chemical and microbial degradation of ten selected pesticides in aquatic systems. In: *Residue Reviews* 45:113–114, Gunther, F. A. and Gunther, J. D. (Eds.). Springer-Verlag, New York, 1973.

31. Jensen, S. The PCB story. *Ambio* 1:123–131, 1972.

32. Anon. Destruction of chemical wastes: ID stage 3. *Kem. Tidskr.* 87:78–79, 1975.

33. Karlsson, L. and Rosen, E. On the thermal destruction of polychlorinated biphenyls (PCB). Some equilibrium considerations. *Chem. Scr.* 1:61–63, 1971.

34. Whitmore, F. C. *Destruction of Polychlorinated Biphenyls in Sewage Sludge During Incineration.* U.S. NTIS PB Rep. 258162, 81 pp., Springfield, Virginia, 1976.

35. Tamura, T., Ohta, Y., and Miyazaki, A. Treatment for chlorinated organic compounds. *Japanese Patent #76-111,468,* Oct. 1, 1976.

36. Ackerman, D., Clausen, J., Johnson, R., Tobias, R., and Zee, C. *Destroying Chemical Wastes in Commercial Scale Incinerators.* U.S. NTIS PB Rep. **PB-270897,** 173 pp., Springfield, Virginia, 1977.

37. Ota, E., Inoue, S., and Otani, S. Decomposition of polychlorinated biphenyls into carbon and hydrogen chloride using molten salt. *Nippon Kagaku Kaishi:* 1407–1409, 1977.

38. Fenn, R. J., Krantz, K. W., and Stuart, J. D. Anodic oxidation of two polychlorinated biphenyls. *J. Electrochem. Soc.* 123:1643–1647, 1976.

39. Stuart, J. D., Keenan, R. R., Fenn, R. J., Jensen, R. G., and Pudelkiewicz, W. J. Degradation of PCB's as studied by oxidative electrochemistry. *Prepr. Pap. Nat. Meet. Div. Water Air Waste Chem., Am. Chem. Soc.* 12:80–84, 1972.

40. Zal'Kind, Yu. S. and Belikova, M. V. Structure of several polychloro derivatives of biphenyl. *J. Gen. Chem. U.S.S.R.* 8:1918–1921, 1938.

41. Choi, P. S. K., Nack, H., and Flinn, J. E. Distribution of polychlorinated biphenyls in an aerated biological oxidation wastewater treatment system. *Bull. Environ. Contam. Toxicol.* 11:12–17, 1974.

42. Tucker, E. S., Saeger, V. W., and Hicks, O. Activated sludge primary biodegradation of polychlorinated biphenyls. *Bull. Environ. Contam. Toxicol.* 14:705–713, 1975.

43. Wong, P. T. S. and Kaiser, K. L. E. Bacterial degradation of polychlorinated biphenyls II. Rate studies. *Bull. Environ. Contam. Toxicol.* 13:249–256, 1975.

44. Kaiser, K. L. E. and Wong, P. T. S. Bacterial degradation of polychlorinated biphenyls. I. Identification of some metabolic products from Aroclor 1242. *Bull. Environ. Contam. Toxicol.* 11:291–296, 1974.

45. Ahmed, M. and Focht, D. D. Oxidation of polychlorinated biphenyls by *Achromobacter pCB. Bull. Environ. Contam. Toxicol.* 10:70–72, 1973.

46. Ahmed, M. and Focht, D. D. Degradation of polychlorinated biphenyls by two species of *Achromobacter. Can. J. Microbiol.* 19:47–52, 1973.

47. Furukawa, K. and Matsumura, F. Microbial metabolism of polychlorinated biphenyls. Studies on the relative degradability of polychlorinated biphenyl components by *Alkaligenes* sp. *J. Agric. Food Chem.* 24:251–256, 1976.

48. Baxter, R. A., Gilbert, P. E., Lidgett, R. A., Mainprize, J. H., and Vodden, H. A. The degradation of polychlorinated biphenyls by micro-organisms. *Sci. Total Environ.* 4:53–61, 1975.

49. Lunt, D. and Evans, W. C. The microbial metabolism of biphenyl. *Biochem. J.* **118**:54P–55P, 1970.
50. Neu, H. J. and Ballschmiter, K. Degradation of chlorinated aromatics: microbiological degradation of polychlorinated biphenyls (PCB). II. Biphenylol as a metabolite of PCB. *Chemosphere* **6**:419–423, 1977.
51. Ballschmiter, K., Unglert, Ch., and Neu, H. J. Degradation of chlorinated aromatic substances: microbiological degradation of polychlorinated biphenyls (PCB). III. Chlorinated benzoic acid as a metabolite of PCB. *Chemosphere* **6**:51–56, 1977.
52. Sayler, G. S., Shon, M., and Colwell, R. R. Growth of an estuarine *Pseudomonas* sp. on polychlorinated biphenyl. *Microb. Ecol.* **3**:241–255, 1977.
53. Nissen, T. V. Stability of PCB in soil (polychlorinated biphenyls). *Tiddskr. Planteavl.* **77**:533–539, 1973.
54. Vockel, D. and Korte, F. Ecological chemistry. LXXX. Microbial degradation of dieldrin and 2,2'-dichlorobiphenyl. *Chemosphere* **3**:177–182, 1974.
55. Statesir, W. A. Explosive reactivity of organics and chlorine. *Chem. Eng. Prog.* **69**(4):52–54, 1973.
56. Tatsukawa, R. and Wakimoto, T. Pollution analysis. Determination of polychlorinated biphenyl in soil. *Kogai Bunseki Shishin* **6**:45–56, 1972.
57. Farwell, S. O., Beland, F. A., and Geer, R. D. Reduction pathways of organohalogen compounds. Part II. Polychlorinated biphenyls. *Electroanal. Chem. Interfacial Electrochem.* **61**:315–324, 1975.
58. LaPierre, R. B., Biron, E., Wu, D., Guczi, L., and Kranich, W. L. *Catalytic Conversion of Hazardous and Toxic Chemicals: Catalytic Hydrodechlorination of Polychlorinated Pesticides and Related Substances.* U.S. NTIS PB Rep. 262804, 184 pp., Springfield, Virginia, 1977.
59. Bailin, L. J., Hertzler, B. L., and Oberacker, D. A. Development of microwave plasma detoxification process for hazardous wastes—Part 1. *Environ. Sci. Technol.* **12**:673–679, 1978.
60. Furukawa, K., Tonomura, K., and Kamibayashi, A. Effect of chlorine substitution on the biodegradability of polychlorinated biphenyls. *Appl. Environ. Microbiol.* **35**:223–227, 1978.
61. Rosenblatt, G., Mozzon, D., Guilford, N. G. H., and Thomas, G. H. S. Polychlorinated biphenyl source emission strengths from municipal incineration and electrical component filling systems. *Proc. Int. Clean Air Congr., 4th:* 637–640, 1977.
62. Ahling, B. and Lindskog, A. Thermal destruction of PCB and hexachlorobenzene. *Sci. Total Environ.* **10**:51–59, 1978.

ETHERS, OXIDES, AND EPOXIDES

DIEPOXYBUTANE (1464-53-5: UNSPECIFIED ISOMER)

Degradation Technique	Remarks	Reference
Hydrolysis	Rapidly hydrolyzed at pH of rat stomach. No details.	1
Hydrolysis	Slowly hydrolyzed to give erythritol or threitol. No details.	2
Hydrolysis Reaction with nucleophiles	Many epoxides were studied, including much detail for diepoxybutane. In 24 h, $37°C$: 15.5% reacted with water, 30% with 0.05 N HOAc, but 100% reacted with 0.5 N NaOH or with $0.25 M S_2O_3^=$ (or $0.5 M I^-$) in 0.05 N acetic acid.	3
Reaction with nucleophiles	Rate constants were determined at pH 7, $37°C$.	4

Diepoxybutane

1. Van Duuren, B. L., Langseth, L., Orris, L., Teebor, G., Nelson, N., and Kuschner, M. Carcinogenicity of epoxides, lactones, and peroxy compounds. IV. Tumor response in epithelial and connective tissue in mice and rats. *J. Natl. Cancer Inst.* **37**:825–838, 1966.
2. *Int. Agency Res. Cancer Monogr.* **11**:116, Lyon, France, 1976.
3. Ross, W. C. J. The reactions of certain epoxides in aqueous solutions. *J. Chem. Soc.*: 2257–2272, 1950.
4. Van Duuren, B. L. and Goldschmidt, B. M. Carcinogenicity of epoxides, lactones, and peroxy compounds. III. Biological activity and chemical reactivity. *J. Med. Chem.* **9**:77–79, 1966.

p-DIOXANE (123-91-1)

Degradation Technique	Remarks	Reference
Oxidation	Flash point: 12°C. Autoignition temperature: 180°C. Auto-oxidation gives peroxides which may be hazardous when concentrated (distillation).	1
Oxidation	Forms explosive peroxides in air, especially in the presence of moisture.	2
Oxidation	The stability of dioxane and other glycol ethers was studied in the range $70-130^{\circ}$C.	3
Oxidation	A kinetic study of oxidation at $50-95^{\circ}$C.	4
Oxidation	Oxidation by H_2O_2 to form HCHO was catalyzed by Cu^{+2} complexes of substituted amino acids.	5
Oxidation	Liquid dioxane was completely converted to the di- and monoformates of ethanediol when heated for two days in the presence of a slow stream of O_2 and a Rh and Li catalyst.	6
Oxidation	Electrolysis in an aqueous solution of 0.5 M Na_2SO_4 produced glyoxal and HCHO.	7
Oxidation	Hazardous reactions cited. First aid and disposal of spills are described.	8
Photo-decomposition	A study of the mechanism of dioxane photolysis at 185 nm in the presence of N_2O.	9
Photo-decomposition	A study of the products formed during the photolysis of liquid dioxane at 147 and 185 nm.	10
Photo-decomposition	Two isomeric dimers and two isomeric alcohols were formed slowly during UV irradiation of liquid dioxane.	11
Photo-decomposition	Nine previously unreported products were identified or postulated as being formed during UV irradiation of liquid dioxane.	12
Photo-decomposition	The $T_{1/2}$ in air at 27°C was about 3.4 hr in the presence of NO with UV intensity equivalent to 2.6 times that of sunlight; 32 other organic compounds were tested.	13

p-DIOXANE (123-91-1)
(continued)

Degradation Technique	Remarks	Reference
Photo-decomposition	Pulsed flashes from a ruby laser decomposed gaseous dioxane into C_2H_4, CO, H_2, and a trace of HCHO. Only 4% conversion was obtained under the conditions used.	14
Photo-decomposition	147 nm photolysis of gaseous dioxane resulted in mainly C_2H_4 and HCHO; only 1.5% conversion of dioxane occurred under the conditions used.	15
Ionizing radiation	Only 4% degradation occurred during radiation with a pulsed laser beam at 694 nm. Auto-oxidation at $25°C$, initiated by ^{60}Co irradiation, produced HCHO and glycol monoformate.	16

p-Dioxane

1. *Handbook of Reactive Chemical Hazards:* 410, Bretherick, L. (Ed.). CRC Press, Cleveland, Ohio, 1975.
2. *Int. Agency Res. Cancer Monogr.* **11**:247, Lyon, France, 1976.
3. Vlasov, G. M., Redoshkin, B. A., Baklanov, N. V., and Ganyushkina, N. K. Thermooxidative stability of monoalkyl glycol ethers. *Khim. Elementoorg Soedin* **4**:112–113, 1976.
4. Rakhmankulov, D. L., Martem'yanov, V. S., Agisheva, S. A., Vdovin, V. A., and Zlotskii, S. S. Kinetics and mechanism of the initiated oxidation of 1,4-dioxacyclanes. *Khim. Geterotsikl Soedin:* 1190–1194, 1975.
5. Sychev, A. Ya. and Biu Ngok Tho. Oxidation of dioxane by hydrogen peroxide in the presence of complexes of copper (II) with N-substituted amino acids. *Izv. Vyssh. Uchebn. Zaved., Khim. Khim. Tekhnol.* **13**:1054–1055, 1970.
6. Henbest, H. B. and Trocha-Grimshaw, J. Aspects of catalysis. VI. Oxidations of sulphoxides and dioxan by dioxygen. *J. Chem. Soc., Perkin Trans.* **1**:607–608, 1974.
7. Goosen, A., Laue, H. A. H., and Roudnick, J. Anodic oxidation. The cleavage of aliphatic ethers. *J. S. Afr. Chem. Inst.* **23**:200–202, 1970.
8. *Hazards in the Chemical Laboratory, 2nd ed.:* 248–249, Muir, G. D. (Ed.). The Chemical Society, London, 1977.
9. Von Sonntag, C. and Bandmann, H. Solvated electrons from excited (λ 185 nm) p-dioxane. *J. Phys. Chem.* **78**:2181–2182, 1974.

10. Kiwi, J. The photochemistry of liquid 1,4-dioxane at 184.8 nm and 147.0 nm. *J. Photochem.* **7**:237–249, 1977.
11. Mazzocchi, P. H. and Bowen, M. W. Photolysis of dioxane. *J. Org. Chem.* **40**:2689–2690, 1975.
12. Houser, J. J. and Sibbio, B. A. Liquid-phase photolysis of dioxane. *J. Org. Chem.* **42**:2145–2151, 1977.
13. Dilling, W. L., Bredeweg, C. J., and Tefertiller, N. B. Organic photochemistry. Simulated atmospheric photodecomposition rates of methylene chloride, 1,1,1-trichloroethane, trichlorethylene, tetrachloroethylene, and other compounds. *Environ. Sci. Technol.* **10**:351–356, 1976.
14. Watson, E. Jr. and Parrish, C. F. Laser induced decomposition of 1,4-dioxane. *J. Chem. Phys.* **54**:1427–1428, 1971.
15. Hentz, R. R. and Parrish, C. F. Photolysis of gaseous 1,4-dioxane at 1470 Å. *J. Phys. Chem.* **75**:3899–3901, 1971.
16. Decker, C. and Marchal, J. Use of oxygen-18 in the study of mechanism of the degradative autooxidation of 1,4-dioxane at 25°C. *C. R. Acad. Sci., Ser. C* **270**:1102–1105, 1970.

4-NITROQUINOLINE-1-OXIDE (56–57–5)

Degradation Technique	Remarks	Reference
Photo-decomposition	The photodynamic toxicity of 4-NQO and related compounds was studied with *Paramecium caudatum*. Free radical formation occurred in the presence of O_2 and UV radiation.	1
Reaction with thiols	The nitro group was replaced by the –SH of cysteine or glutathione at 37°C, pH 7.	2
Reaction with $Na_2 S_2 O_3$	The mutagenic activity of 4-NQO was destroyed by treatment with an equal volume of 5% $Na_2 S_2 O_3$. 4-NQO was stable for at least six months at 4°C in phosphate buffer, pH 7.	3
Chemical	A review of the chemical properties of 4-NQO and its derivatives, including nucleophilic substitutions and reduction of the nitro group, deoxygenation of the N-oxide group, and miscellaneous reactions.	4

4-NQO: 4-nitroquinoline-1-oxide

4-Nitroquinoline-1-oxide

1. Nagata, C., Fujii, K., and Epstein, S. S. Photodynamic activity of 4-nitro-quinoline-1-oxide and related compounds. *Nature* 215:972–973, 1967.
2. Endo, H. On the relation between carcinogenic potency of 4-nitroquinoline N-oxides and the reactivity of their nitro-groups with SH-compounds. *Gann* 49:151–156, 1958.
3. Bal, J., Kajtaniak, E. M., and Pieniazek, N. J. 4-Nitroquinoline-1-oxide: a good mutagen for *Aspergillus nidulans. Mutat. Res.* 56:153–156, 1977.
4. Kawazoe, Y. Chemical properties. In: *Chemistry and Biological Actions of 4-Nitroquinoline-1-oxide:* 3–16, Endo, H., Ono, T., and Sugimura, T. (Eds.). *Recent Results in Cancer Research* 34, Springer-Verlag, New York, 1971.

HYDRAZINES

HYDRAZINES*

Degradation Technique	Remarks	Reference
Thermal	Rate constants were determined during very low pressure pyrolysis. Apparatus and theory were covered in previous publications (see General Procedures #46 and 47).	1
Thermal	The products of several methyl hydrazines were determined after thermal decomposition in the presence or absence of a catalyst.	2
Chemical	Physical and chemical properties were given, including reactions that may be useful for the degradation of hydrazines.	3
Oxidation	A study of the effects of droplet size, O_2 concentration, and temperature as related to combustion of propellants.	4
Oxidation	HCHO was formed during partial degradation of methyldrazine derivatives by treatment with hexacyanoferrate.	5
Oxidation	Methylhydrazine derivatives formed H_2O_2 when auto-oxidized in aqueous solution in the presence of O_2. The effects of pH, buffer concentration, and free radical acceptors were studied. Products were identified.	6
Oxidation	This dissertation included a study of the oxidation of hydrazines by lead tetraacetate and by phosgene.	7
Oxidation	p-Benzoquinone oxidized the hydrazine moiety quantitatively to N_2 in basic solutions. Basis for analysis.	8
Oxidation	The hydrazine moiety was oxidized quantitatively to N_2 in basic solutions containing different inorganic oxidants. Basis for analysis.	9

*See also hydrazine, methylhydrazine, and dimethylhydrazine.

HYDRAZINES
(continued)

Degradation Technique	Remarks	Reference
Oxidation	The hydrazine moiety was oxidized quantitatively to N_2 in acidic solutions containing $KMnO_4$ or $K_2Cr_2O_7$ plus Cu^{+2}. Other oxidizing agents were included in the study as a basis for analysis.	10
Oxidation	Electrochemical oxidation was studied at a platinum electrode in dimethyl sulfoxide. The products were identified.	11

Hydrazines

1. Golden, D. M., Solly, R. K., Gac, N. A., and Benson, S. W. Very low-pressure pyrolysis. VII. The decomposition of methylhydrazine, 1,1-dimethylhydrazine, 1,2-dimethylhydrazine, and tetramethylhydrazine. Concentrated deamination and dehydrogenation of methylhydrazine. *Int. J. Chem. Kinet.* **4**:433–448, 1972.
2. Martignoni, P., Duncan, W. A., Murfee, J. A. Jr., Nappier, H. A., and Phillips, J. *Thermal and Catalytic Decomposition of Methyldrazines.* U.S. NTIS AD Rep. **749262**, 24 pp., Springfield, Virginia, 1972.
3. Raphaelian, L. A. Hydrazine and its derivatives. In: *Kirk-Othmer Encyclopedia of Chemical Technology, 2nd ed.* **11**:164–196. John Wiley & Sons, New York, 1966.
4. Allison, C. B. and Faeth, G. M. Decomposition and hybrid combustion of hydrazine, MMH and UDMH as droplets in a combustion gas environment. *Combust. Flame* **19**:213–226, 1972.
5. Weitzel, G., Schneider, F., Fretzdorff, A. M., Durst, J., and Hirschmann, W. D. Studies on the mechanism of the cytostatic action of methylhydrazine II. *Hoppe-Seyler's Z. Physiol. Chem.* **348**:433–442, 1967.
6. Berneis, K., Kofler, M., Bollag, W., Zeller, P., Kaiser, A., and Langemann, A. Peroxidative effect of tumor inhibiting methylhydrazine compounds. *Helv. Chim. Acta* **46**:2157–2167, 1963.
7. Stone, D. M. Hydrazine oxidations. *Diss. Abstr. Int. B* **36**:3397, 1976.
8. Hassan, S. S. M. and Zaki, M. T. M. Microdetermination of the hydrazine function: a new gasometric method based on oxidation with benzoquinone. *Microchem. J.* **15**:470–474, 1970.

9. Hassan, S. S. M. Gasometric microdetermination of hydrazine compounds by oxidation with some inorganic oxidants in acidic media. *Anal. Chim. Acta* 54:185–187, 1971.
10. Hassan, S. S. M. Microgasometric determination of the hydrazine function by oxidation with some inorganic oxidants in acidic media. *Anal. Chim. Acta* 54:185–187, 1971.
11. Michlmayr, M. and Sawyer, D. T. Electrochemical oxidation of hydrazine and of the dimethylhydrazines in dimethylsulfoxide at a platinum electrode. *J. Electroanal. Chem. Interfacial Electrochem.* 23:375–385, 1969.

1,1-DIMETHYLHYDRAZINE* (57-14-7)

Degradation Technique	Remarks	Reference
Oxidation	Flammable: flash point is $-15°C$. Powerful reducing agent and fuel. No details.	1
Oxidation	Flammable. Vapor ignites spontaneously in the presence of oxidizing agents. Relatively stable in the dark and cold. No details.	2
Oxidation	Reaction in acid solution with $HgSO_4$ released one methyl group as HCHO. Methylhydrazine remained.	3
Oxidation	An aqueous solution of UDMH was refluxed in air for 20 hr at $90°C$ to release one methyl group as HCHO.	4
Oxidation	Treatment with selenium dioxide in dilute H_2SO_4 for 30 min at $50°C$ released one methyl group as HCHO.	5
Oxidation	A flotation method for wastewater decontamination was described, using air oxidation catalyzed by activated charcoal. In some cases, Cl_2 was added.	6
Oxidation	A German patent, including modification of the procedures described in reference #6.	7
Oxidation	A study of the quantitative formation of tetramethyltetrazene at $0°C$ by the oxidation of UDMH with I_2 or Br_2 at neutral or weakly basic pH, and with KIO_3 or $KBrO_3$ at acid pH followed by neutralization.	8

*See also hydrazines.

1,1-DIMETHYLHYDRAZINE (57-14-7)
(continued)

Degradation Technique	Remarks	Reference
Oxidation	Further study of the dimerization of UDMH after oxidation in acid solutions of $KBrO_3$.	9
Oxidation	Reacted with $CuCl_2$ in aqueous solution at pH 4 and $0°C$ to form a product which rapidly decomposed when stored dry in air (one sample burned spontaneously!) Product formed tetramethyltetrazene when made alkaline.	10
Oxidation	Anodic oxidation on Pt in acid electrolyte gave the diazenium salt.	11
Oxidation	A kinetic study of the electrochemical oxidation of UDMH on Au electrodes in dilute H_2SO_4.	12
Oxidation	An electrochemical process was studied in acetonitrile.	13
Oxidation	Chemical oxidation was studied with acid solutions of $KBrO_3$ or Ce^{+4}. Reaction mechanisms were compared with those for electrochemical oxidation.	14
Oxidation	Ignites violently with oxidizing agents such as N_2O_4, H_2O_2, and HNO_3.	15
Ozonation	A kinetic study of the oxidation of aqueous solutions of UDMH by O_3. Products were N_2, CO_2, and tetramethyltetrazene.	16
Ozonation	Treatment with O_3 on an Al_2O_3 catalyst produced CO_2, N_2, and water.	17
Reaction with enyne ethers	Reacted in aqueous acid to give 1,5-dimethylpyrazole.	18

UDMH: unsymmetrical DMH = 1,1-dimethylhydrazine

1,1-Dimethylhydrazine

1. *Handbook of Reactive Chemical Hazards:* 330, Bretherick, L. (Ed.). CRC Press, Cleveland, Ohio, 1975.
2. *Int. Agency Res. Cancer Monogr.* 4:137, Lyon, France, 1974.
3. Preussmann, R., Hengy, H., and Von Hodenberg, A. A new photometric analytical method for 1,1-dialkylhydrazines. *Anal. Chim. Acta* 42:95–99, 1968.
4. Sutton, N. V. Spectrophotometric determination of unsymmetrical dimethylhydrazine employing chromotropic acid. *Anal. Chem.* 36:2120–2121, 1964.
5. Lynch, V. P. Method for determining 'Alar' (B–995) residues in apples. *J. Sci. Food Agric.* 20:13–14, 1969.
6. Höke, B. and Wittbold, H.-A. Catalytic oxidation of dissolved nitrite, cyanide, UDMH and hydrazine. *Wasser Luft. Betr.* 13:250–252, 1969.
7. Höke, B. Decontaminating and purifying sewage containing hydrazine, dimethylhydrazine, and nitrogen tetroxide. *German Patent #1,517, 634,* Dec. 21, 1972.
8. McBride, W. R. and Kruse, H. W. Alkylhydrazines. I. Formation of a new diazo-like species by the oxidation of 1,1-dialkylhydrazines in solution. *J. Am. Chem. Soc.* 79:572–576, 1957.
9. McBride, W. R. and Bens, E. M. Alkylhydrazines. III. Dimerization of certain substituted 1,1-dialkyldiazenes to tetraalkyltetrazenes. *J. Am. Chem. Soc.* 81:5546–5550, 1959.
10. Boehm, J. R., Balch, A. L., Bizot, K. F., and Enemark, J. H. Oxidation of 1,1-dimethylhydrazine by cupric halides. The isolation of a complex of 1,1-dimethyldiazene and a salt containing the 1,1,5,5-tetramethylformazanium ion. *J. Am. Chem. Soc.* 97:501–508, 1975.
11. Karabinas, P. and Heitbaum, J. The anodic oxidation of hydrazine derivatives on platinum in acid electrolytes. III. Dimethylhydrazine. *J. Electronal. Chem. Interfacial Electrochem.* 76:247–255, 1977.
12. Eisner, U. and Zommer, N. Anodic oxidation of hydrazine and its derivatives. II. The oxidation of 1,1-dimethylhydrazine (DMH) on gold electrodes in acid solution. *J. Electroanal. Chem. Interfacial Electrochem.* 30:433–441, 1971.
13. Cauquis, G., Chabaud, B., and Genies, M. Electrochemical oxidation of 1,1-dimethylhydrazine and trimethylhydrazine in acetonitrile. *J. Electroanal. Chem. Interfacial Electrochem.* 40:6–10, 1972.
14. Atkinson, T. V. and Bard, A. J. Electron spin resonance studies of cation radicals produced during oxidation of methylhydrazines. *J. Phys. Chem.* 75:2043–2048, 1971.
15. *Hazards in the Chemical Laboratory, 2nd ed.:* 241, Muir, G. D. (Ed.). The Chemical Society, London, 1977.

16. Lysenko, T. F., Atyaksheva, L. F., Strakhov, B. V., and Emel'yanova, G. I. Study of the kinetics and mechanism of oxidation of 1,1-dimethylhydrazine by ozone in an aqueous solution. *Zh. Fiz. Khim.* 49:3131–3134, 1975.
17. Emel'yanova, G. I., Lysenko, T. F., Atyaksheva, L. F., and Strakhov, B. V. Study of the kinetics and mechanism of the heterogeneous oxidation of 1,1-dimethylhydrazine by ozone. *Zh. Fiz. Khim.* 51:85–88, 1977.
18. Belyaeva, A. N., Maretina, I. A., and Petrov, A. A. Reaction of enyne ethers and their substituted hetero analogs with unsymmetrical dialkylhydrazines. *Zh. Org. Khim.* 8:651, 1972.

1,2-DIMETHYLHYDRAZINE* (540-73-8)

Degradation Technique	Remarks	Reference
Oxidation	Flash point is less than $23°C$.	1
Oxidation	Flammable. Relatively stable in the dark and cold. Traces of heavy metal catalyzed rapid dehydrogenation to give azomethane. No details.	2
Reaction with $S_2 Cl_2$	Dichlorodisulfane reacted with SDMH to form tetramethylcyclotetrasulfurdihydrazide and other products.	3

SDMH: symmetrical DMH = 1,2-dimethylhydrazine

*See also hydrazines.

1,2-Dimethylhydrazine

1. *Handbook of Reactive Chemical Hazards:* 330, Bretherick, L. (Ed.). CRC Press, Cleveland, Ohio, 1975.
2. *Int. Agency Res. Cancer Monogr.* 4:145, Lyon, France, 1974.
3. Lingmann, H. and Linke, K.-H. The reaction of hydrazine and 1,2-dimethylhydrazine with dichlorodisulfane. *Z. Naturforsch., Teil B* 26:1207–1209, 1971.

HYDRAZINE* (302-01-2)

Degradation Technique	Remarks	Reference
Oxidation	Flammable. Explodes if air is present during distillation. Affected by UV and metal ion catalysts. No details.	1
Oxidation	Flash point is $38°C$. Autoignition temperatures are $23°C$ on a rusty surface, $132°C$ on iron, $156°C$ on stainless steel. Once ignited, it will burn without air or oxidant. Other warnings cited.	2
Oxidation	Oxidation with I_2, $KBrO_3$, or $KMnO_4$ was complete in aqueous solutions. Basis for analysis.	3
Oxidation	Rapid volumetric analyses were based on oxidation by HIO_3, I_2, Br_2, or $HOCl$.	4
Oxidation	A kinetic study of the Cu^{+2}-catalyzed oxidation of hydrazine by H_2O_2, in the absence of air, to form N_2 and water.	5
Oxidation	The stoichiometry of oxidation by acidic solutions of $KMnO_4$ and $K_2Cr_2O_7$ was studied at $30°C$.	6
Oxidation	The stoichiometry of oxidation by HNO_2 was studied.	7
Oxidation	Dichlorodisulfane oxidized an ethereal solution of hydrazine to form N_2.	8
Oxidation	The oxidation of hydrazine by iodine at alkaline pH was presented as a laboratory experiment.	9
Oxidation	$K_3Fe(CN)_6$ oxidized hydrazine at alkaline pH in aqueous methanol. The reaction rate was affected by the methanol concentration and the addition of certain neutral salts.	10
Oxidation	A kinetic study was made of the oxidation of hydrazine, as a copper complex, by peroxydisulfate at $35°C$. The effects of pH and ionic strength were determined.	11

*See also hydrazines.

HYDRAZINE (302-01-2)
(continued)

Degradation Technique	Remarks	Reference
Oxidation	A Raney Ni catalyst was used for the decomposition of hydrazine in low-concentration solutions.	12
Oxidation	Hydrazine reacted with H_2O_2 in aqueous solution to form N_2 and water. The reaction required the presence of trace metal ions and was inhibited by EDTA.	13
Oxidation	Aqueous or caustic solutions of hydrazine were stable for 90 days at 20–70°C in Pyrex glass when air was excluded. The hydrazine diminished with time when the solutions were partially exposed to air.	14
Oxidation	The oxidation by $HClO_4$ was studied in the presence of a Mo^{+6} catalyst.	15
Oxidation	Quantitative oxidation to N_2 and water occurred in acid solution in the presence of $KMnO_4$ and NaF with $CuSO_4$ as catalyst. Basis for analysis.	16
Oxidation	A cobalt chelate catalyzed the oxidation of hydrazine by oxygen at pH 11.5 in aqueous solution.	17
Oxidation	Quantitative oxidation occurred in 5 min by $K_2Cr_2O_7$ in 0.2–0.8 N HCl. Basis for analysis.	18
Oxidation	A kinetic study was made of oxidation by Tl^{+3} in H_2SO_4. The effects were determined of varying concentrations of NaCl, Na_2SO_4, Tl^{+3}, $KHSO_4$, H_2SO_4, and $N_2H_4 \cdot 2H_2SO_4$.	19
Oxidation	Various reagents were described for the quantitative oxidation of hydrazine.	20
Oxidation	Oxidation by metaperiodate was the basis for analysis.	21
Oxidation	A kinetic study was made of the oxidation by peroxodiphosphate to form N_2 and $H_2PO_4^-$.	22

HYDRAZINE (302-01-2)
(continued)

Degradation Technique	Remarks	Reference
Oxidation	The hydrogenation of various olefins was strongly catalyzed by Cu ion. Diimide was the intermediary, its oxidation leading to the formation of N_2.	23
Oxidation	The relative rates of hydrogenation by hydrazine were determined with various unsaturated acids.	24
Oxidation	Power plant effluents were treated with O_2 on an activated charcoal column.	25
Oxidation	The rate of oxidation of hydrazine in power plant effluents was studied with and without the addition of coal ash.	26
Oxidation	Reaction with chlorinated lime was used in removing hydrazine from power plant effluents.	27
Oxidation	A flotation method for wastewater decontamination was described, using air oxidation catalyzed by activated charcoal.	28
Oxidation	Electrochemical oxidation occurred in liquid NH_3 electrolytes on Pt and other electrodes.	29
Oxidation	Hydrazine was completely degraded into N_2 and H_2 on a Pt electrode in alkaline solution at 20–80°C.	30
Oxidation	Electrochemical oxidation on Pt electrodes was studied in acid solution.	31
Oxidation	Electrochemical oxidation on Au electrodes was studied in acid solutions.	32
Oxidation	Hydrazine (diamide) was oxidized to diimide by sodium metaperiodate. The diimide was used for reducing olefins in the same solution in which it was generated.	33
Oxidation Reaction with nitrosalicylaldehyde	Hydrazine was oxidized in a few days in water depending on hardness, organic matter, etc. The reaction with nitrosalicylaldehyde to form an insoluble aldazine was the basis for analysis.	34

HYDRAZINE (302-01-2)
(continued)

Degradation Technique	Remarks	Reference
Oxidation Thermal	Decomposition of hydrazine in the presence of several catalysts, with or without the application of electric current, occurred mainly without N-N bond rupture.	35
Thermal	A kinetic study was made of the decomposition of hydrazine between $1000°$ and $1400°K$. The reaction proceeded mainly as $N_2H_4 \rightarrow NH_3 + NH$; the NH reacted with added NO to form N_2O+H.	36
Thermal	Pyrolysis at $900°C$ completely degraded hydrazine to form mostly NH_3 and some N_2. Decomposition was incomplete at lower temperatures.	37
Thermal	Pyrolysis of hydrazine gas was catalyzed on a fused-silica surface at low pressure and high temperature to form N_2, NH_3, and H_2.	38
Thermal	Hydrazinium ions catalyzed the decomposition of hydrazine at $153-201°C$.	39
Thermal	Hydrazine was adsorbed on a tungsten film and its decomposition was studied at various temperatures. NH_3, N_2, and H_2 were produced by heterogenous catalysis. Data for other surfaces were included.	40
Thermal	Hydrazine was adsorbed on a film of molybdenum and its decomposition to NH_3, H_2, and N_2 was studied at various temperatures.	41
Thermal	Degradation of hydrazine adsorbed on ZnO started at the N-H bond and later involved the N-N bond.	42
Thermal	A kinetic study at low temperatures ($40-90°C$) with the formation of N_2 on $Bi(MoO_4)_3$ and MoO_3 catalysts.	43
Thermal	Degradation occurred at $139-174°C$ while adsorbed on Ni filaments.	44
Thermal	Degradation occurred at $146-290°C$ while adsorbed on Fe filaments.	45

HYDRAZINE (302-01-2)
(continued)

Degradation Technique	Remarks	Reference
Thermal	The kinetics of decomposition were studied at $120-220°C$ on Pd foil and membrane.	46
Reaction with HNO_2	N-nitrosohydrazine formed and decomposed to HN_3 at high acidity, and to NH_3 and N_2O at low acidity.	47
Reaction with cis-butene-1,4-diones	Pyridazines or N-aminopyrroles were formed.	48
Reaction with $LiBH_4$	The reaction was used as a source of H_2: $N_2H_4 \cdot 2HCl + 2\ LiBH_4 \rightarrow 2BN + 7H_2 + 2LiCl$.	49
Reduction	The reaction was studied in acid, neutral, and alkaline media. In neutral solution, hydrazine oxidized $Ru(NH_3)_6{}^{2+}$ to $Ru(NH_3)_6{}^{3+}$.	50
Photo-decomposition	The flash photolysis of hydrazine gas was studied.	51
Photo-decomposition	Various inorganic compounds sensitized hydrazine photo-oxidation in aqueous solution. In acid medium, the products were NH_3, N_2, and water; in neutral or weakly alkaline solution, N_2 and water were produced.	52
Photo-decomposition	The kinetics of hydrazine decomposition by UV light (206 nm) were studied in the presence and absence of ethylene or dimethylmercury.	53
Ionizing radiation	A study of the mechanism of decomposition of hydrazine gas by an electron beam.	54
Chemical	A detailed review of reactions of commercial value, with 384 references. Includes a section on hazards and methods for handling hydrazine.	55
	First aid and disposal of spills are described.	56
Thermal	Hydrazine was decomposed at $400-800°C$ and the products were added to flue gases containing NO_x, which was reduced to N_2 and water.	57

Hydrazine

1. The Merck Index, 9th ed.: entry #4653, Windholz, M., Buavari, S., Stroumtsos, L. Y., and Fertig, M. N. (Eds.). Merck and Co., Rahway, New Jersey, 1976.

2. Handbook of Reactive Chemical Hazards: 809, Bretherick, L. (Ed.). CRC Press, Cleveland, Ohio, 1975.

3. Kolthoff, I. M. The volumetric analysis of hydrazine by the iodine, bromate, iodate and permanganate methods. J. Am. Chem. Soc. 46:2009–2016, 1924.

4. Bray, W. C. and Cuy, E. J. The oxidation of hydrazine. I. The volumetric analysis of hydrazine by the iodic acid, iodine, bromine, and hypochlorous acid methods. J. Am. Chem. Soc. 46:858–875, 1924.

5. Wellman, C. R., Ward, J. R., and Kuhn, L. P. Kinetics of the oxidation of hydrazine by hydrogen peroxide, catalyzed by hydrated copper (II). J. Am. Chem. Soc. 98:1683–1684, 1976.

6. Prasad, R. K. and Kumar, A. Oxidation of hydrazine with acid permanganate and dichromate. Part II. J. Indian Chem. Soc. 50:612–613, 1973.

7. Prasad, R. K. and Kumar, A. Oxidation of hydrazine by nitrous acid. Part III. J. Indian Chem. Soc. 50:572–574, 1973.

8. Lingmann, H. and Linke, K.-H. The reaction of hydrazine and 1,2-dimethylhydrazine with dichlorodisulfane. Z. Naturforsch., Teil B 26:1207–1209, 1971.

9. Cooper, J. N. and Ramette, R. W. The oxidation of hydrazine by basic iodine solutions. J. Chem. Educ. 46:872–873, 1969.

10. Jindal, V. K., Agrawal, M. C., and Mushran, S. P. Oxidation of hydrazine by alkaline ferricyanide in water-methanol mixtures. Z. Naturforsch., Teil B 25:188–190, 1970.

11. Swaroop, R. and Gupta, Y. K. Kinetics of the oxidation of copper-hydrazine complex by peroxydisulphate. Indian J. Chem. 9:361–364, 1971.

12. Voznesenskii, N. M. Decomposition of hydrazine in low-concentration solutions. Tr. Mosk. Energ. Inst.: 79–81, 1976.

13. Kuhn, L. P. and Wellman, C. Metal-ion Catalyzed Oxidation of Hydrazine with Hydrogen Peroxide. U.S. NTIS AD Rep. 746956, 15 pp., Springfield, Virginia, 1972.

14. Bott, T. R. and Rassoul, G. A. R. Pyrex glass and the decomposition of hydrazine in solution. Chem. Ind. (London): 39, 1972.

15. Koltunov, V. S., Tikhonov, M. F., and Kuperman, A. Ya. Oxidation of hydrazine by perchloric acid catalyzed by molybdenum. Zh. Fiz. Khim. 50:2859–2862, 1976.

16. Issa, I. M., Issa, R. M., Hammam, A. M., and Mahmoud, M. R. Oxidation with potassium permanganate in presence of fluoride. Volumetric and potentiometric determination of hydrazine. J. Indian Chem. Soc. 53:698–704, 1976.

17. Cookson, D. J., Smith, T. D., Boas, J. F., Hicks, P. R., and Pilbrow, J. R. Electron spin resonance study of the autooxidation of hydrazine, hydroxylamine, and cysteine catalyzed by the cobalt (II) chelate complex of 3, 10, 17, 24-tetrasulphophthalocyanine. *J. Chem. Soc., Dalton Trans.:* 109-114, 1977.

18. Mahmoud, M. R., Issa, I. M., Ghandour, M. A., and Hammam, A. M. Determination of hydrazine using potassium dichromate as oxidizing agent. *Indian J. Chem.* 14A:70-71, 1976.

19. Srinivasan, V. S. and Venkatasubramanian, N. Oxidation of hydrazine, phenylhydrazine and substituted phenylhydrazines by thallium (III)—substituent effects and mechanism. *Indian J. Chem.* 15A:115-117, 1977.

20. Audrieth, L. and Ogg, B. *The Chemistry of Hydrazine:* 153-162. John Wiley & Sons, New York, 1951.

21. Kaushik, R. L., Vermani, O. P., and Prosad, R. Determination of hydrazine, methylhydrazine, semicarbazide and hexacyanoferrate (II) using periodate. *Indian J. Chem.* 14A:1022-1023, 1976.

22. Kapoor, S. and Gupta, Y. K. Kinetics and mechanism of oxidations by peroxodiphosphate-IV. *J. Inorg. Nucl. Chem.* 39:1019-1021, 1977.

23. Corey, E. J., Mock, W. L., and Pasto, D. J. Chemistry of diimide. Some new systems for the hydrogenation of multiple bonds. *Tetrahedron Lett.:* 347-352, 1961.

24. Hünig, S. and Müller, R.-H. Reductions with diimide. II. *Angew. Chem.* 74:215-216, 1962.

25. Akol'zin, P. A. and Kostrikina, E. Yu. Contact oxidation of hydrazine by atmospheric oxygen dissolved in water. *Primen Gidrazina Teploenerg Ustanovkakh Elektrostn:* 23-31, 1973.

26. Panich, R. U., Naryshkin, D. G., Voznesenskii, N. M., and Prokof'ev, G. I. Oxidation of hydrazine in waste waters in a hydraulic ash removal system. *Teploenergetika:* 59-61, 1977.

27. Gronskii, R. K., Ivanov, E. N., Bodnar, Yu. F., Maklakova, V. P., and Gruzdeva, A. F. Decontamination of spent anticorrosion solutions. *Elektr. Stn.:* 75-76, 1973.

28. Höke, B. and Wittbold, H.-A. Catalytic oxidation of dissolved nitrite, cyanide, UDMH and hydrazine. *Wasser Luft. Betr.* 13:250-252, 1969.

29. Milles, M. H. and Kellett, P. M. Electrode oxidation of hydrazine and related compounds in liquid ammonia electrolytes. *J. Electrochem. Soc.* 117:60-65, 1970.

30. Vitvitskaya, G. V. Mechanism of electrode reactions of hydrazine in an alkaline medium. *Elektrokhimiya* 6:1234-1237, 1970.

31. Harrison, J. A. and Khan, Z. A. Oxidation of hydrazine on platinum in acid solution. *J. Electroanal. Chem. Interfacial Electrochem.* 28:131-138, 1970.

32. Eisner, U. and Gileadi, E. Anodic oxidation of hydrazine and its derivatives. I. Oxidation of hydrazine on gold electrodes in acid solutions. *J. Electroanal. Chem. Interfacial Electrochem.* **28**:81–92, 1970.
33. Hoffman, J. M. Jr. and Schlessinger, R. H. Sodium metaperiodate: a mild oxidizing agent for the generation of di-imide from hydrazine. *J. Chem. Soc., Chem. Commun.:* 1245–1246, 1971.
34. Slonim, A. R. and Gisclard, J. B. Hydrazine degradation in aquatic systems. *Bull. Environ. Contam. Toxicol.* **16**:301–309, 1976.
35. Arnolds, K., Heitbaum, J., and Veilstich, W. Investigations on the rupture of the N-N bond within the anodic oxidation and catalytic decomposition of hydrazine. *Z. Naturforsch., Teil A* **29**:359–360, 1974.
36. Meyer, E. and Wagner, H. Gg. On the mechanism of the thermal decomposition of hydrazine. *Z. Phys. Chem.* **89**:329–331, 1974.
37. Harke, H. P., Schüller, D., and Drews, C. J. Pyrolysis of maleic hydrazide and hydrazine. *Z. Lebensm. Unters.-Forsch.* **153**:163–169, 1973.
38. Stein, S. E., Benson, S. W., and Golden, D. M. Very low-pressure pyrolysis (VLPP) of hydrazine, ethanol, and formic acid on fused silica. *J. Catal.* **44**:429–438, 1976.
39. Rubtsov, Yu. I. and Manelis, G. B. Kinetics of the homogeneous catalytic liquid-phase decomposition of hydrazine. *Zh. Fiz. Khim.* **43**:2972–2973, 1969.
40. Cosser, R. C. and Tompkins, F. C. Heterogeneous decomposition of hydrazine on tungsten films. *Trans. Faraday Soc.* **67**:526–544, 1971.
41. Contaminard, R. C. A. and Tompkins, F. C. Heterogeneous decomposition of hydrazine on molybdenum films. *Trans. Faraday Soc.* **67**:545–555, 1971.
42. Tsivenko, V. I. and Myasnikov, I. A. Chemisorption of NH_2 radicals on oxide semiconductors in connection with the catalytic decomposition of nitrogen-containing substances. *Probl. Kinet. Katal.* **14**:198–201, 1970.
43. Santacesaria, E., Giuffre, L., and Gelosa, D. Kinetics of hydrazine decomposition at low temperature on reduced molybdates. *Riv. Combust.* **25**:62–67, 1971.
44. Fatu, D. and Segal, E. Kinetic study of the decomposition of hydrazine on nickel filaments. *An. Univ. Bucuresti Chim.* **19**:121–125, 1970.
45. Fatu, D. and Segal, E. Kinetics of the decomposition of hydrazine on iron filaments. *An. Univ. Bucuresti Chim.* **19**:61–66, 1970.
46. Khomenko, A. A. and Apel'bum, L. O. Study of the kinetics of the catalytic decomposition of hydrazine vapors on palladium. *Kinet. Mater.–Vses. Konf. Kinet. Katal. Reakts, 2nd* **1**:143–152, 1975.
47. Perrott, J. R., Stedman, G., and Uysal, N. Kinetic and product study of the reaction between nitrous acid and hydrazine. *J. Chem. Soc., Dalton Trans.:* 2058–2064, 1976.

48. Rio, G. and Lecas-Nawrocka, A. Formation of N-aminopyrroles by reaction of hydrazine with cis-butene-1,4-diones. Photooxidation of 1-amino-tetraphenylpyrrole. *Bull. Soc. Chim. Fr.:* 1723–1727, 1971.
49. Beckert, W. F., Dengel, O. H., and McKain, R. W. Generating hydrogen. *U.S. Patent #3,931,395,* Jan. 6, 1976.
50. Bottomley, F. Reactions of hydrazine with ruthenium compounds. *Can. J. Chem.* 48:351–355, 1970.
51. Arvis, M., Devillers, C., Gillois, M., and Curtat, M. Isothermal flash photolysis of hydrazine. *J. Phys. Chem.* 78:1356–1360, 1974.
52. Shevchenko, G. P., Pushkareva, T. M., and Sviridov, V. V. Sensitization of hydrazine photooxidation in an aqueous solution by lead and titanium oxides and hydroxides. *Zh. Fiz. Khim.* 44:546, 1970.
53. Schurath, U. and Schindler, R. N. The photolysis of hydrazine at 2062Å in the presence of ethylene. *J. Phys. Chem.* 74:3188–3194, 1970.
54. Bubert, H. and Froben, F. W. The decomposition of ammonia and hydrazine by electron impact. *J. Phys. Chem.* 75:769–771, 1971.
55. Byrkit, G. D. and Michalek, G. A. Hydrazine in organic chemistry. *Ind. Eng. Chem.* 42:1862–1875, 1950.
56. *Hazards in the Chemical Laboratory, 2nd ed.:* 277–278, Muir, G. D. (Ed.). The Chemical Society, London, 1977.
57. Azuhata, S., Kikuchi, H., Akimoto, H., Hishinuma, Y., Arikawa, Y., and Oshima, R. Noncatalytic reduction of nitrogen oxides in flue gases. *Japanese Patent # 78-72772,* June 28, 1978.

METHYLHYDRAZINE* (60-34-4)

Degradation Technique	Remarks	Reference
Microsomal Oxidation	Rat liver microsomes produced methane; more rapid nonenzymatic degradation occurred at higher temperatures ($>37°C$) by vapor phase decomposition in air.	1
Oxidation	Oxidation of the vapor in air produced mainly N_2 and some CH_4 (at 22–24°C). $T_{1/2}$ was 34 min in a glass container, but the reaction was complete in 10 min in a polyethylene container due to surface catalysis.	2
Oxidation	Ignites spontaneously with strong oxidizing agents. No details.	3

*See also hydrazines.

METHYLHYDRAZINE (60-34-4)
(continued)

Degradation Technique	Remarks	Reference
Oxidation	Flash point is $23°C$. Autoignition temperature is $196°C$.	4
Oxidation	A study was made of the effects of pressure, temperature, and reactant proportions for the spontaneous ignition (explosive combustion) of methylhydrazine gas and O_2.	5
Oxidation	The reaction mechanism was studied during oxidation by ceric ammonium sulfate or $KBrO_3$ in acid solution.	6
Oxidation	The oxidation mechanism was studied with ceric ion in acid solution.	7
Oxidation	Oxidation by metaperiodate was the basis for analysis.	8
Oxidation	Anodic oxidation at a Pt electrode in acid solution produced CH_3OH and N_2.	9
Oxidation	Oxidation was studied on Hg electrodes in alkaline solution.	10

Methylhydrazine

1. Prough, R. A., Wittkop, J. A., and Reed, D. J. Evidence for the hepatic metabolism of some monoalkylhydrazines. *Arch. Biochem. Biophys.* **131**: 369-373, 1969.
2. Vernot, E. H., MacEwen, J. D., Geiger, D. L., and Haun, C. C. The air oxidation of monomethyl hydrazine. *J. Am. Ind. Hyg. Assoc.* **28**:343-347, 1967.
3. *The Merck Index, 9th ed.:* entry #5954, Windholz, M., Buavari, S., Stroumtsos, L. Y., and Fertig, M. N. (Eds.). Merck and Co., Rahway, New Jersey, 1976.
4. *Handbook of Reactive Chemical Hazards:* 254, Bretherick, L. (Ed.). CRC Press, Cleveland, Ohio, 1975.
5. Gray, P. and Sherrington, M. E. Self-heating and spontaneous ignition in the combustion of gaseous methylhydrazine. *J. Chem. Soc., Faraday Trans. I* **70**:740-751, 1974.
6. Atkinson, T. V. and Bard, A. J. Electron spin resonance studies of cation

radicals produced during oxidation of methylhydrazines. *J. Phys. Chem.* 75:2043–2048, 1971.

7. Knoblowitz, M., Miller, L., Morrow, J. I., Rich, S., and Scheinbart, T. Oxidation of methylhydrazine by cerium (IV) in acid media. *Inorg. Chem.* 15:2847–2849, 1976.

8. Kaushik, R. L., Vermani, O. P., and Prosad, R. Determination of hydrazine, methylhydrazine, semicarbazide & hexacyanoferrate (II) using periodate. *Indian J. Chem.* 14A:1022–1023, 1976.

9. Karabinas, P. and Heitbaum, J. The anodic oxidation of hydrazine derivatives at platinum in acid electrolytes. II. Methylhydrazine. *J. Electroanal. Chem. Interfacial Electrochem.* 76:235–246, 1977.

10. Eisner, U. and Zemer, Y. Anodic oxidation of hydrazine and its derivatives. III. Oxidation of methylhydrazine on mercury electrodes in alkaline solution. *J. Electroanal. Chem. Interfacial Electrochem.* 34:81–89, 1972.

PROCARBAZINE
(671–16–9: FREE BASE)
(366–70–1: HYDROCHLORIDE)

Degradation Technique	Remarks	Reference
Thermal Oxidation Photo- decomposition	A review of the properties of procarbazine hydrochloride. It melts at about $233°C$ with decomposition. Auto-oxidation of solutions is catalyzed by Mn^{+2} and Cu^{+2}. It is very sensitive to UV light.	1
Oxidation	Partial dehydrogenation to yield HCHO occurred during treatment with hexacyanoferrate.	2
Oxidation	The effect of metal ions on the oxidation of procarbazine was studied at pH 7. Catalysis by Cu^{+2} was markedly inhibited by the addition of Ti^{+4}, whereas catalysis by Mn^{+2} was markedly stimulated by Ti^{+4}. The toxicity and fate of the diazo product was not discussed.	3
Oxidation	The auto-oxidation of methylhydrazine derivatives (such as procarbazine) gave rise to diazo derivatives, which were relatively rapidly converted to hydrazones. The latter hydrolyzed to form methylhydrazine.	4
	Possible degradation products were tested for carcinogenicity in mice. The azo and hydrazone derivatives induced pulmonary tumors.	5

Procarbazine

1. Rucki, R. J. Procarbazine hydrochloride. *Anal. Profiles Drug Subst.* 5:403–427, 1976.
2. Weitzel, G., Schneider, F., Fretzdorff, A. M., Durst, J., and Hirschmann, W.-D. Studies on the mechanism of the cytostatic action of methylhydrazine. II. *Hoppe-Seyler's Z. Physiol. Chem.* 348:433–442, 1967.
3. McCue, J. P. and Kennedy, J. H. Oxidation of procarbazine in the presence of Ti(IV). *Bioinorg. Chem.* 7:5–21, 1977.
4. Berneis, K., Kofler, M., Bollag, W., Zeller, P., Kaiser, A., and Langemann, A. Peroxidative effect of tumor inhibiting methylhydrazine compounds. *Helv. Chim. Acta* 46:2157–2167, 1963.
5. Kelly, M. G., O'Gara, R. W., Yancey, S. T., Gadekar, K., Botkin, C., and Oliverio, V. T. Comparative carcinogenicity of N-isopropyl-α-(2-methyl-hydrazine)-p-toluamide·HCL (procarbazine hydrochloride), its degradation products, other hydrazines, and isonicotinic acid hydrazide. *J. Natl. Cancer Inst.* 42:337–344, 1969.

NITROGEN MUSTARDS

CHLORAMBUCIL (305-03-3)

Degradation Technique	Remarks	Reference
Hydrolysis	At 37°C in 0.025 N NaOH (pH 11.5), hydrolysis was complete in 120 min. At 60°C, it was complete in 30 min. No significant hydrolysis occurred at 5°C in 24 hr.	1
Hydrolysis	39% was hydrolyzed in 30 min when refluxed with 50% aqueous acetone.	2
Hydrolysis	The hydrolysis was inhibited by the addition of serum albumin to Tris buffer, pH 7, at 37°C.	3
Hydrolysis Reaction with 4-(p-nitrobenzyl)-pyridine	$T_{1/2}$ was 30 min at 37°C, pH 7.4. This was inhibited by many proteins and other polymers. $T_{1/2}$ was 18 hr in 6 N HCl at 105–110°C. A blue-colored product resulted when 4-(p-nitrobenzyl)-pyridine was heated for 5 min at 100°C with chlorambucil.	4

Chlorambucil

1. Linford, J. H. Some interactions of nitrogen mustards with constituents of human blood serum. *Biochem. Pharmacol.* 8:343–357, 1961.
2. Redel, J., Brouilhet, H., Bazely, N., Jouanneau, M., Calando, Y., and Delbarre, F. The chemical reactivity and biological properties of the homologues of chlorambucil. *C. R. Acad. Sci., Ser. D* 275:2433–2436, 1972.
3. Paulaityte, N. and Konstantinavicius, K. Reactivity of the alkylating agents hisphen, B-100, and chlorambucil in aqueous solutions and biological substrates. *Liet. T. S. R. Mokslu. Akad. Darb., Ser. C* (1):111–117, 1977.
4. Hopwood, W. J. and Stock, J. A. The effect of macromolecules upon the rates of hydrolysis of aromatic nitrogen mustard derivatives. *Chem.-Biol. Interact.* 4:31–39, 1971/72.

URACIL MUSTARD (66-75-1)

Degradation Technique	Remarks	Reference
Thermal	Decomposed at 206°C.	1
Thermal Hydrolysis	Decomposed at 200°C. Unstable in water or acid solutions. No details.	2
Microbial	Tritium-labeled uracil mustard was converted into bacterial pyrimidines.	3

Uracil Mustard

1. Lyttle, D. A. and Petering, H. G. 5-Bis-(2-chlorethyl)-aminouracil, a new anti-tumor agent. *J. Am. Chem. Soc.* **80**:6459–6460, 1958.
2. *Int. Agency Res. Cancer Monogr.* **9**:235, Lyon, France, 1975.
3. Wacker, A., Kirschfeld, S., and Träger, L. On the mechanism of action of thymine analog cytostatics in bacteria. *Naturwissenschaften* **53**:257–258, 1966.

ALIPHATIC HALIDES

ALIPHATIC HALIDES*

Degradation Technique	Remarks	Reference
Chemical	Reactivity of polychlorinated aliphatic compounds was included in this review with 105 references.	1
Microbial	EDB and DBCP were included in studies of reductive dehalogenation by soil microbes. Pure cultures were not isolated; soil was present. EDB→ethylene + Br$^-$ (complete in two months); DBCP→propanol + Br$^-$ + Cl$^-$ (63% in one month).	2
Microbial	Merely stated that EDB and DBCP "are readily degraded."	3
Microbial Photo-decomposition	Microbial degradation of alkyl halides was considered not to be significant. Photo-oxidation in the atmosphere was the principal mechanism for their destruction.	4
Photo-decomposition Hydrolysis	A review article including: VC, EDB, CHCl$_3$, CCl$_4$, BCME, and CMME; 242 references.	5
Dehalogenation	DBCP was one of several alkyl halides that reacted rapidly with Fe^{++}-porphyrins at room temperature.	6
Dehalogenation	Vicinal dihalides were reduced by Cr^{+2} to corresponding olefins in high yields. DBCP and EDB were included.	7
Oxidation	Waste gases were incinerated with an O$_2$-containing gas in the presence of a NiO catalyst at 100–200°C.	8
Oxidation	Waste gases were oxidized at 50–300°C in the presence of a Co$_3$O$_4$ catalyst.	9

*See also specific compounds.

ALIPHATIC HALIDES
(continued)

Degradation Technique	Remarks	Reference
Oxidation	Halogenated organic compounds, especially those with 1–4 C-atoms, were removed from air by oxidation over Ru or Pt catalysts at about 350–375°C.	10

BCME:	bis(chloromethyl)ether	DBCP:	1,2-dibromo-3-chloropropane
CMME:	chloromethyl methyl ether	EDB:	ethane (1,2-dibromo-)
		VC:	vinyl chloride

Aliphatic Halides

1. Bonse, G. and Henschler, D. Chemical reactivity, biotransformation and toxicity of polychlorinated aliphatic compounds. *C. R. C. Crit. Rev. Toxicol.* 4:395–409, 1976.
2. Castro, C. E. and Belser, N. O. Biodehalogenation. Reductive dehalogenation of the biocides ethylene dibromide, 1,2-dibromo-3-chloropropane, and 2,3-dibromobutane in soil. *Environ. Sci. Technol.* 2:779–783, 1968.
3. Beckman, H., Crosby, D. G., Allen, P. T., and Mourer, C. The inorganic bromide content of foodstuffs due to soil treatment with fumigants. *J. Food Sci.* 32:138–140, 1967.
4. McConnell, G., Ferguson, D. M., and Pearson, C. R. Chlorinated hydrocarbons and the environment. *Endeavour* 34:13–18, 1975.
5. Fishbein, L. Industrial mutagens and potential mutagens. I. Halogenated aliphatic derivatives. *Mutat. Res.* 32:267–308, 1976.
6. Castro, C. E. The rapid oxidation of iron (II) porphyrins by alkyl halides. A possible mode of intoxication of organisms by alkyl halides. *J. Am. Chem. Soc.* 86:2310–2311, 1964.
7. Kray, W. C. Jr. and Castro, C. E. The cleavage of bonds by low-valent transition metal ions. The homogeneous dehalogenation of vicinal dihalides by chromous sulfate. *J. Am. Chem. Soc.* 86:4603–4608, 1964.
8. Lavanish, J. M. and Sare, E. J. Catalytic oxidation of C_2-C_4 halogenated hydrocarbons. *U.S. Patent #4,039,623*, Aug. 2, 1977.
9. Sare, E. J. and Lavanish, J. M. Treatment of a gas stream containing a chlorinated or brominated C_2-C_4 hydrocarbon. *German Patent #2,700,236*, July 21, 1977.

10. Yang, K., Scamehorn, J. F., Reedy, J. D., and Lindberg, R. C. Decomposition of halogenated organic compounds. *German Patent #2,640,906,* March 17, 1977.

CARBON TETRACHLORIDE* (56-23-5)

Degradation Technique	Remarks	Reference
Oxidation	Incineration yielded CO_2, HCl, $COCl_2$, and Cl_2. No details.	1
Oxidation	Oxidation over a zeolite catalyst removed 84–90% of CH_2Cl_2 and CCl_4 from waste gases.	2
Oxidation	Oxidation over zeolite catalyst gave HCl or Cl_2, depending upon the temperature and type of catalyst. Other alkyl chlorides were included in the study.	3
Oxidation	Oxidation in the presence of a Cu-zeolite catalyst gave Cl_2 and HCl at temperatures around $500°C$. Phosgene was also produced at lower temperatures. Other organic chloride waste products behaved similarly.	4
Microwave discharge	Decomposition (80–90%) to Cl_2, HCl, H_2, C, and CO occurred in 10–20 min in a high-frequency electrodeless discharge.	5
Physico-chemical	Physical and chemical properties and reactions were given. Many degradation reactions were described, some of which yielded toxic products (e.g., $COCl_2$) or explosions.	6
Chemical	CCl_4 rapidly halogenated ketones and sulfones at $25°C$ in the presence of powdered KOH-*t*-butanol. Alcohols were oxidized by CCl_4 under these conditions.	7
	Hazardous reactions cited.	8
	Hazardous reactions cited. First aid and handling of spills were described.	9

*See also aliphatic halides.

Carbon Tetrachloride

1. *Int. Agency Res. Cancer Monogr.* 1:53, Lyon, France, 1972.
2. Ivanova, G. A., Doronina, L. M., Eshenbakh, L. F., Lobanov, V. M., Filippova, T. E., and Bogdan, N. P. Detoxification of gas emissions from production of a movie film base. *Prom. Sanit. Ochistka Gazov* (5):26–27, 1976.
3. Doronina, L. M., Ivanova, G. A., and Abramova, G. V. Zeolites as catalysts of the exhaustive oxidation of chloroorganic substances. *Zh. Prikl. Khim.* **50**:1820–1823, 1977.
4. Hyatt, D. E. Low temperature catalytic oxidation of chlorinated organic compounds to recover chlorine values. *U.S. Patent #3,989,806*, Nov. 2, 1976.
5. Zimina, I. D., Maksimov, A. I., and Svettsov, V. I. Decomposition of carbon tetrachloride molecules in a high-frequency electrodeless discharge. *Izv. Vyssh. Uchebn. Zaved. Khim. Khim. Tekhnol.* **20**:1099, 1977.
6. Hardie, D. W. F. Carbon tetrachloride. In: *Kirk-Othmer Encyclopedia of Chemical Technology, 2nd ed.* **5**:128–139. John Wiley & Sons, New York, 1964.
7. Kolb, V. M. The unique properties of powdered potassium hydroxide-*t*-butyl alcohol as a reagent, and as medium for chlorinations with CCl_4: a mechanistic study of the reactions and reactivities of ketones, sulfones, and alcohols. *Diss. Abstr. Int. B* 37:4466, 1977.
8. *Handbook of Reactive Chemical Hazards:* 219, Bretherick, L. (Ed.). CRC Press, Cleveland, Ohio, 1975.
9. *Hazards in the Chemical Laboratory, 2nd ed.:* 181, Muir, G. D. (Ed.). The Chemical Society, London, 1977.

CHLOROFORM* (67-66-3)

Degradation Technique	Remarks	Reference
Oxidation	May explode with acetone in the presence of KOH or $Ca(OH)_2$. Other hazards were cited.	1
Oxidation	Chlorinated hydrocarbons were degraded to CO_2 and HCl at low temperatures in the presence of a Pt catalyst. $CHCl_3$ was 97.6% degraded at 460°C.	2
Oxidation Photo-decomposition Thermal Reduction	Described physical and chemical properties and many degradative reactions.	3

*See also aliphatic halides.

CHLOROFORM (67–66–3)
(continued)

Degradation Technique	Remarks	Reference
Photo-decomposition	Irradiation at 365.5 nm at $30°C$ in the presence of Cl_2 and O_2 produced HCl and $COCl_2$.	4
Reaction with ketones	In alkali, $R_2CO + CHCl_3$ yielded $R_2C(OH)CCl_3$, which could be hydrolyzed to give $R_2C(OH)COOH$.	5
Reaction with sodium azide	Two min at $-80°C$ yielded 4,4,4-trichlorobu-tyronitrile.	6
Hydrolysis	In sea water. Very questionable results due to evaporation; at best very inefficient.	7
	Hazardous reactions cited. First aid and handling of spills were described.	8

Chloroform

1. *Handbook of Reactive Chemical Hazards:* 226, Bretherick, L. (Ed.). CRC Press, Cleveland, Ohio, 1975.
2. Anon. Catalytic destruction of chlorinated hydrocarbons. *British Patent #1,485,375*, Sept. 8, 1977.
3. Hardie, D. W. F. Chloroform. In: *Kirk-Othmer Encyclopedia of Chemical Technology, 2nd ed.* 5:119–127. John Wiley & Sons, New York, 1964.
4. Sanhueza, E. The chlorine atom sensitized oxidation of $HCCl_3$, HCF_2Cl and HCF_3. *J. Photochem.* 7:325–334, 1977.
5. Lurie, A. P. Ketones. In: *Kirk-Othmer Encyclopedia of Chemical Technology, 2nd ed.* 12:121. John Wiley & Sons, New York, 1967.
6. Bikales, N. M. Cyanoethylation. In: *Kirk-Othmer Encyclopedia of Chemical Technology, 2nd ed.* 6:642. John Wiley & Sons, New York, 1965.
7. Jensen, S. and Rosenberg, R. Degradability of some chlorinated aliphatic hydrocarbons in sea water and sterilized water. *Water Res.* 9:659–661, 1975.
8. *Hazards in the Chemical Laboratory, 2nd ed.:* 192–193, Muir, G. D. (Ed.). The Chemical Society, London, 1977.

1,2-DIBROMO-3-CHLOROPROPANE* (96-12-8)

Degradation Technique	Remarks	Reference
Microbial	Soil metabolism studies indicated that DBCP was degraded by microorganisms.	1
Microbial	DBCP was readily dissipated and caused an increase in the number of soil bacteria.	2
Microbial	About 90% was destroyed in nine weeks with about 10% moisture at $21-24°C$. Soil micro-organisms were assumed to be responsible for the degradation.	3
Microbial	DBCP could still be recovered from soil 40 weeks after application to field plots.	4
Microbial	Soil-water cultures dehalogenated DBCP to form n-propanol, Cl^-, and Br^-. About 63% degradation occurred in three weeks at room temperature.	5
Thermal	When heated for 30 min at $180°C$, DBCP was converted from a liquid to a yellow powder with loss of Br and/or Cl atoms. Other pesticides were included in this study.	6
Oxidation	Modified pyrolysis $(+O_2)$ at $900°C$ yielded CO, CO_2, HCl, and Cl_2; 19 other pesticides included.	7
Oxidation	Almost complete destruction was achieved at $600°C$ in a muffle furnace.	8
Oxidation	Incineration at $900°C$ produced CO, CO_2, HCl, and Cl_2.	9
	Guidelines for the control of exposure to DBCP. Gives physical properties, including flash point (above $175°C$), and toxicity data.	10
Hydrolysis	Stable in neutral or acidic media. Hydrolyzed in alkali to give 2-bromoallyl alcohol. No details.	11

DBCP: 1,2-dibromo-3-chloropropane

*See also aliphatic halides.

1,2-Dibromo-3-chloropropane

1. Jaramillo, R. and Blasco, M. Effect on the soil metabolism of the nematicide 1,2-dibromo-3-chloropropane. *Turrialba* 23:480–482, 1973.
2. Naidu, S. M. Pesticide residues and their effects on microbial activities following massive disposal of pesticides in the soil. *Diss. Abstr. Int. B* 33: 2894, 1973.
3. Hodges, L. R. and Lear, B. Efficacy of 1,2-dibromo-3-chloropropane for control of *Meloidogyne javanica* as influenced by concentration, exposure time and rate of degradation. *J. Nematol.* 5:249–253, 1973.
4. Hodges, L. R. Distribution and persistence of 1,2-dibromo-3-chloropropane in soil. *Diss. Abstr. Int. B* 32:4968, 1972.
5. Castro, C. E. and Belser, N. O. Biodehalogenation. Reductive dehalogenation of the biocides ethylene dibromide, 1,2-dibromo-3-chloropropane, and 2,3-dibromobutane in soil. *Environ. Sci. Technol.* 2:779–783, 1968.
6. Stojanovic, B. J., Hutto, F., Kennedy, M. V., and Shuman, F. L. Jr. Mild thermal degradation of pesticides. *J. Environ. Qual.* 1:397–401, 1972.
7. Kennedy, M. V., Stojanovic, B. J., and Shuman, F. L. Jr. Analysis of decomposition products of pesticides. *J. Agric. Food Chem.* 20:341–343, 1972.
8. Kennedy, M. V., Stojanovic, B. J., and Shuman, F. L. Jr. Chemical and thermal methods for disposal of pesticides. In: *Residue Reviews* 29:89–104, Gunther, F. A. and Gunther, J. D. (Eds.). Springer-Verlag, New York, 1969.
9. Kennedy, M. V., Stojanovic, B. J., and Shuman, F. L. Jr. Chemical and thermal aspects of pesticide disposal. *J. Environ. Qual.* 1:63–65, 1972.
10. Madsen, F. Occupational Safety and Health Administration guidelines for control of exposure to 1,2-dibromo-3-chloropropane. *Occup. Saf. Health Rep.* 6:434–438, 1977.
11. *Int. Agency Res. Cancer Monogr.* 15:139, Lyon, France, 1977.

ETHYLENE DIBROMIDE* (106–93–4: 1,2-ISOMER)

Degradation Technique	Remarks	Reference
Reaction with nucleophiles	Rate constants were determined at 20° and 37°C. Included other alkylating compounds.	1
Oxidation	EDB was completely converted to KBr by oxidation for 1 hr at room temperature in an alkaline solution of K_2CrO_4. Basis for colorimetric analysis.	2
Oxidation	Oxidation in a catalytic furnace produced Br^- Basis for analysis.	3
Oxidation	Elemental Br_2 was recovered by treating EDB with O_2 at 600–800°C in the presence of a Cr_2O_3 catalyst.	4
Hydrolysis	Treatment with NaOH in a solution of ethanol and benzene liberated Br^-. Basis for analysis.	5
Hydrolysis	Heating with ethanolamine for 30 min at 90°C completely hydrolyzed EDB to Br^-. Basis for analysis.	6
Hydrolysis	Ethylene glycol was prepared by autoclaving EDB with KOAc in water for 1 hr at 160°C under N_2. Reaction was not complete.	7
Microbial	Soil-water cultures dehalogenated EDB almost completely to give C_2H_4 and Br^- in eight weeks at room temperature.	8
Photodecomposition	Sensitive to light. No details.	9

EDB: ethylene dibromide

*See also aliphatic halides

Ethylene Dibromide

1. Ehrenberg, L., Osterman-Golkar, S., Singh, D., and Lundqvist, U. On the reaction kinetics and mutagenic activity of methylating and β-halogenoethylating gasoline additives. *Radiat. Bot.* 15:185–194, 1974.
2. Rangaswamy, J. R., Vijayashankar, Y. N., and Muthu, M. Colorimetric

method for the determination of ethylene dibromide residues in grains and
air. *J. Assoc. Off. Anal. Chem.* **59**:1262–1265, 1976.

3. Wade, P. Determination of fumigants. XXII. Photometric determination of
brominated hydrocarbon fumigants as inorganic bromide. *J. Sci. Food Agric.*
3:390–393, 1952.
4. Davis, R. A. and Tigner, R. G. Catalytic recovery of bromine from organic
bromides. *U.S. Patent #3,705,010,* Dec. 5, 1972.
5. Kennett, B. H. and Huelin, F. E. Determination of ethylene dibromide in
fumigated fruit. *J. Agric. Food Chem.* **5**:201–203, 1957.
6. Sinclair, W. B. and Crandall, P. R. Determination of ethylene dibromide in
liquid and gas phases by the use of monoethanolamine. *J. Econ. Entomol.*
40:80–82, 1952.
7. Okitsu, H. and Hirose, I. Alkylene glycols. *Japanese Patent #77-42,807,*
April 4, 1977.
8. Castro, C. E. and Belser, N. O. Biodehalogenation. Reductive dehalogenation of the biocides ethylene dibromide, 1,2-dibromo-3-chloropropane,
and 2,3-dibromobutane in soil. *Environ. Sci. Technol.* **2**:779–783, 1968.
9. *The Merck Index, 9th ed.:* entry #3732, Windholz, M., Buavari, S., Stroumtsos, L. Y., and Fertig, M. N. (Eds.). Merck and Co., Rahway, New Jersey,
1976.

VINYL CHLORIDE* (75–01–4)

Degradation Technique	Remarks	Reference
Oxidation	Combustion gases were analyzed. HCl was found to be the main source of danger in a VC fire, but $COCl_2$, CO, and CO_2 were also produced.	1
Oxidation	Almost 100% degradation to HCl occurred with 1 ml H_2/min and 60 ml CO/min at 1200°K. Basis for analysis.	2
Oxidation	Polyperoxide forms in air (can explode). A 20–30% NaOH solution destroys the peroxide. Discharge of the vapor and spray under pressure creates static electricity, which can result in an explosion.	3
Oxidation	Treatment with O_2 at 20–300°C in the presence of a catalyst removed VC from waste gases.	4
Oxidation	Air containing 5500 ppm VC was heated to about 376°C in the presence of a Ru catalyst	5

*See also aliphatic halides.

VINYL CHLORIDE (75-01-4)
(continued)

Degradation Technique	Remarks	Reference
	to give 2 ppm VC in the flue gas. The Cl in VC was converted to Cl_2 and HCl.	
Oxidation	Air containing 5000 ppm VC was heated at $450°C$ in the presence of a Mg/Cr catalyst for 1.2 sec to give 99.7% decomposition. Other organic Cl compounds were also decomposed.	6
Oxidation	The VC content of moist gas was reduced from 141 ppm to 2.7 ppm by treatment with O_3 at $29°C$.	7
Oxidation	A marked reduction in VC content was obtained by treating waste gas and water with $KMnO_4$.	8
Oxidation	More than 99% of VC in waste gases was decomposed at $320°C$ in the presence of Cr_2O_3.	9
Oxidation	Air containing 5000 ppm VC was heated at $450°C$ in the presence of a Cr-Cu catalyst for 0.3 sec to give 99% decomposition.	10
Oxidation	A commercial system was described for incinerating VC and other hydrocarbons in waste gases with the recovery of HCl and heat.	11
Oxidation Chlorination	A commercial system was described for decomposing chlorinated hydrocarbons and other products of VC manufacture in waste gases and water. Useful by-products were formed.	12
Oxidation Chlorination	In the presence of Cl_2 and O_2 at $50–60°C$, VC was converted to $ClCH_2COCl$ in good yield by light of wavelengths 330–350 nm.	13
Chlorination	A study of the formation of trichloroethane from VC gas by irradiation at 436 nm in the presence of Cl_2.	14
Oxidation Photo-decomposition	2000 ppm VC gas was completely decomposed by UV irradiation for 30 sec at room temperature in the presence of phosgene and air. A general procedure for decomposing toxic hydrocarbons was described using O_2 or O_3 in the presence of a Cl-containing accelerator and UV light.	15

VINYL CHLORIDE (75-01-4)
(continued)

Degradation Technique	Remarks	Reference
Oxidation Photo-decomposition	The efficient degradation of VC vapor by UV (185 nm) and O_2 or O_3 at ambient conditions of temperature and pressure was described. The method was applied to gaseous hydrocarbons and halogenated or partially oxidized hydrocarbons.	16
Oxidation Photo-decomposition	After 22 hr irradiation by fluorescent lamps with wavelength maximum at 365 nm, 79% of VC gas was degraded and O_3 was produced in the presence of NO and air.	17
Oxidation Photo-decomposition	The VC content of waste gases was reduced from 140 ppm to 0.6 ppm when bubbled through a solution of NaOCl under UV irradiation.	18
Oxidation Photo-decomposition	A kinetic study was made of the oxidation of VC by Cl atoms or O atoms generated by the photolysis of Cl_2 or O_2. Products were determined.	19
Oxidation Photo-decomposition	$T_{1/2}$ for VC gas in air was about 4.3 hr at 27°C in the presence of NO and UV equivalent to 2.6 times that of sunlight; 32 other organic compounds were tested. NO_2 and O_3 were also tested as oxidants.	20
Photo-decomposition	Degradation (80%) was obtained with a VC gas flow of 2 ℓ/min at 0–25 ppm. More efficient degradation was expected if a UV lamp (254 nm) with higher output were used. Basis for analysis.	21
Photo-decomposition	A kinetic study of the decomposition of VC by UV light in the presence of varying concentrations of Cl_2 gas at room temperature. Products were identified.	22
Photo-decomposition	The decomposition of VC vapor during irradia-by a xenon lamp was markedly accelerated by NO. The products were HCHO and HCl.	23

VINYL CHLORIDE (75-01-4)
(continued)

Degradation Technique	Remarks	Reference
Photo-decomposition	A kinetic study of the decomposition of VC and other gaseous chloroethylenes by UV at $25°C$.	24
Photo-decomposition	A kinetic study was made of the effect of UV irradiation on VC gas at various temperatures in the presence of free radical scavengers.	25
Photo-decomposition Ionizing radiation	A kinetic study was made of the gas-phase UV photolysis and radiolysis of VC.	26
Pyrolysis Oxidation	HCl was recovered during pyrolysis in molten KCl at $800°C$. The introduction of O_2 converted the residual organic matter mainly to CO_2.	27
Acetylation	Vinyl acetate was prepared from VC in the presence of O_2, CH_3COOH, and catalytic salts at $100°C$.	28
Chemical Physical	A review giving physical and chemical properties that may be useful for decontamination. Flash point: $-78°C$.	29
Polymerization	Polymerizes in light or in the presence of a catalyst. No details.	30
	Hazards, first aid, and handling of spills are briefly described.	31

VC: vinyl chloride

Vinyl Chloride

1. O'Mara, M. M., Crider, L. B., and Daniel, R. L. Combustion products from vinyl chloride monomer. *J. Am. Indust. Hyg. Assoc.* 32:153–156, 1971.

2. Cedergren, A. and Fredriksson, S. A. Trace analysis for chlorinated hydrocarbons in air by quantitative combustion and coulometric chloride determination. *Talanta* 23:217–223, 1976.

3. *Handbook of Reactive Chemical Hazards:* 293, Bretherick, L. (Ed.). CRC Press, Cleveland, Ohio, 1975.

4. Sare, E. J. and Lavanish, J. M. Reducing the vinyl chloride content of gas streams. *German Patent #2,653,769,* June 8, 1977.

5. Yang, K., Scamehorn, J. F., Reedy, J. D., and Lindberg, R. C. Decomposition of halogenated organic compounds. *German Patent #2,640,906,* March 17, 1977.

6. Kato, H., Mizutani, K., Inoue, H., and Suzuki, H. Catalytic decomposition of organic chlorine compounds in a waste gas. *Japanese Patent #76-69,474,* June 16, 1976.

7. Ban, K., Ito, I., Nagaoka, K., and Takeda, K. Treatment of waste gas containing vinyl chloride. *Japanese Patent #76-10,174,* Jan. 27, 1976.

8. Witenhafer, D. E., Daniels, C. A., and Koebel, R. F. Oxidation of vinylidene halides by permanganates in gaseous or aqueous process streams. *U.S. Patent #4,062,925,* 3 pp., Dec. 13, 1977.

9. Hiraga, H., Kobayashi, S., and Ohta, Y. Removal of polymerizable monomer from waste gas. *Japanese Patent #76-39,566,* April 2, 1976.

10. Kato, H., Mizutani, K., Inoue, H., and Suzuki, H. Catalytic oxidation of organic chlorine compounds. *Japanese Patent #76-22,699,* Feb. 23, 1976.

11. Kiang, Y.-H. Controlling vinyl chloride emissions. *Chem. Eng. Prog.* 72(12): 37–41, 1976.

12. Machida, M. and Tanaka, S. Vinyl chloride monomer production without pollution. *Chem. Econ. Eng. Rev.* 8:31–36, 1976.

13. Shinoda, K. and Konno, K. Reaction of chlorohydrocarbons. I. Chlorine-sensitized photooxidation of vinyl chloride. *Nippon Kagaku Kaishi:* 527–531, 1973.

14. Olbregts, J. Addition of chlorine atom on vinyl chloride. *Bull. Soc. Chim. Belg.* 83:73–76, 1974.

15. Kagiya, T. and Takemoto, K. Removing toxic hydrocarbon derivatives from air by oxidation and ultraviolet light irradiation. *Japanese Patent #76-65,072,* June 5, 1976.

16. Legan, R. W. Photochemical process for decontaminating gaseous or vaporous streams. *U.S. Patent #4,045,316,* Aug. 30, 1977.

17. Cox, R. A., Eggleton, E. J., and Sandalls, F. J. *Photochemical reactivity of vinyl chloride.* U.K. At. Energy Res. Establ., Rep. **7820,** 10 pp., 1974.

18. Ito, I. and Nagaoka, K. Vinyl chloride removal from waste gases. *Japanese Patent #76-23,467*, Feb. 25, 1976.
19. Sanhueza, E. and Heicklen, J. Oxidation of chloroethylene. *J. Phys. Chem.* 79:677–681, 1975.
20. Dilling, W. L., Bredeweg, C. J., and Tefertiller, N. F. Organic photochemistry. Simulated atmospheric photodecomposition rates of methylene chloride, 1,1,1-trichloroethane, trichloroethylene, tetrachloroethylene, and other compounds. *Environ. Sci. Technol.* 10:351–356, 1976.
21. Confer, R. G. A UV-conductivity method for determination of airborne levels of vinyl chloride. *J. Am. Ind. Hyg. Assoc.* 36:491–496, 1975.
22. Kagiya, T. and Takemoto, K. Photooxidative decomposition of vinyl chloride in the presence of chlorine. *Nippon Kagaku Kaishi:* 54–60, 1977.
23. Kanno, S., Nojima, K., Takahashi, K., Iseki, H., Takamori, S., and Takamatsu, K. Studies on the photochemistry of aliphatic halogenated hydrocarbons. II. Photochemical decomposition of vinyl chloride and ethyl chloride in the presence of nitrogen oxides in air. *Chemosphere* 6:509–514, 1977.
24. Müller, J. P. H. and Korte, F. Contributions to ecological chemistry. CXXXVI. Short report on the unsensitized photooxidation of chloroethylenes. *Chemosphere* 6:341–346, 1977.
25. Fujimoto, T., Rennert, A. M., and Wijnen, M. H. J. Primary steps in the photolysis of vinyl chloride. *Ber. Bunsenges. Phys. Chem.* 74:282–286, 1970.
26. Ausloos, P., Rebbert, R. E., and Wijnen, M. H. J. Gas phase for ultraviolet photolysis and radiolysis of vinyl chloride. *J. Res. Natl. Bur. Stand., Sect. A* 77:243–248, 1973.
27. DeBeukelaer, G., Krome, G., Langens, J., Lockefeer, F., and Schaerlaekens, P. Hydrochloric acid manufacture by thermal decomposition of vinyl chloride distillation residues. *German Patent #2,261,795*, July 4, 1974.
28. Tamura, M. and Yasui, A. Vinyl acetate preparation from a vinyl halide. *Japanese Patent #70-14,527*, May 23, 1970.
29. Hardie, D. W. F. Vinyl chloride. In: *Kirk-Othmer Encyclopedia of Chemical Technology, 2nd ed.* 5:171–178. John Wiley & Sons, New York, 1964.
30. *The Merck Index, 9th ed.:* entry #9645, Windholz, M., Buavari, S., Stroumtsos, L. Y., and Fertig, M. N. (Eds.). Merck and Co., Rahway, New Jersey, 1976.
31. *Hazards in the Chemical Laboratory, 2nd ed.:* 430–431, Muir, G. D. (Ed.). The Chemical Society, London, 1977.

NITROFURAN DERIVATIVES

N-[4-(5-NITRO-2-FURYL)-2-THIAZOLYL] FORMAMIDE
(24554-26-5)

Degradation Technique	Remarks	Reference
Thermal	Melts at 295–300°C with decomposition.	1

N-[4-(5-Nitro-2-furyl)-2-thiazolyl] formamide

1. Ertürk, E., Price, J. M., Morris, J. E., Cohen, S., Leith, R. S., Von Esch, A. M., and Crovetti, A. J. The production of carcinoma of the urinary bladder in rats by feeding N-[4-(5-nitro-2-furyl)-2-thiazolyl] formamide. *Cancer Res.* 27:1998–2002, 1967.

SULFONIC ACID DERIVATIVES

BROMOETHYL METHANESULFONATE (4239-10-5)

Degradation Technique	Remarks	Reference
Reaction with CF₃COOH	Various bromoethyl sulfonates gave trifluoroacetyl bromethane when treated with CF₃COOH at 70°C.	1

Bromoethyl Methanesulfonate

1. Shchekut'eva, L. F., Smolina, T. A., Senchenkov, E. P., and Reutov, O. A. Study of trifluoroacetolysis of 2-bromoethyl-l-^{14}C-sulfonates. *Vestn Mosk. Univ. Khim.* **17**:623–624, 1976.

ETHYL METHANESULFONATE (62-50-0)

Degradation Technique	Remarks	Reference
Hydrolysis	The effect of temperature was studied in unbuffered solution: $T_{1/2}$ was 2.7 hr at 50°C. Rate was not affected at pH's of 3, 5, or 7. Products were methanesulfonic acid and ethanol.	1
Hydrolysis	The effects of pH and buffer concentration were studied. $T_{1/2}$ was 9 hr at pH 11 in 0.4 M phosphate buffer at 30°C.	2
Hydrolysis Reaction with nucleophiles	This detailed kinetic study included data for several methanesulfonates. Rate constants were determined at 20°, 25°, and 37°C. Reaction with $S_2O_3{}^{-2}$ was greatest of the compounds tested.	3

Ethyl Methanesulfonate

1. Froese-Gertzen, E. E., Konzak, C. F., Foster, R., and Nilan, R. A. Correlation between some chemical and biological reactions of ethyl methanesulfonate. *Nature* **198**:447–448, 1963.
2. Wickham, I. M., Narayanan, K. R., and Konzak, C. F. Influence of pH and concentration of phosphate buffer on the degradation of alkyl alkanesulphonates. In: *I.A.E.A. Symp. Induced Mutations in Plants, Proc. Symp.:* 153–167, 1969.
3. Osterman-Golkar, S., Ehrenberg, L., and Wachtmeister, C. A. Reaction kinetics and biological action in barley of mono-functional methanesulfonic esters. *Radiat. Bot.* **10**:303–327, 1970.

METHYL METHANESULFONATE (66-27-3)

Degradation Technique	Remarks	Reference
Hydrolysis	A comparison was made of the rates of hydrolysis of methyl sulfonates and halides in water and in dilute NaOH at various temperatures.	1
Hydrolysis Reaction with nucleophiles	This detailed kinetic study included data for several methanesulfonates. Rate constants were determined at $20°$, $25°$, and $37°C$. Reaction with $S_2 O_3{}^{-2}$ was greatest of the compounds tested.	2
Reaction with nucleophiles	A kinetic study was made of reactions with N-Cl- and N-methylbenzenesulfonamide. The rate constant with the former was about five times that with the latter in methanol.	3

Methyl Methanesulfonate

1. Hartman, S. and Robertson, R. E. Nucleophilic displacement of methyl sulphonic esters by hydroxide ion in water. *Can. J. Chem.* **38**:2033–2038, 1960.
2. Osterman-Golkar, S., Ehrenberg, L., and Wachtmeister, C. A. Reaction kinetics and biological action in barley of mono-functional methanesulfonic esters. *Radiat. Bot.* **10**:303–327, 1970.
3. Beale, J. H. The reactivity of N-chloro- and N-methylbenzenesulfonamide anions with methyl methanesulfonate in methanol. *J. Org. Chem.* **37**:3871–3872, 1972.

1,3-PROPANE SULTONE (1120-71-4)

Degradation Technique	Remarks	Technique
Reaction with nucleophiles	Rate constants at 37°C were determined for the reaction with water and more reactive nucleophiles. Included some data on ethyl and methyl methanesulfonates.	1
Reaction with nucleophiles	A review of the chemistry of propane sultone. Hydrolysis was found to be an equilibrium reaction, but with a large excess of water, hydrolysis was essentially complete ($T_{1/2}$ was 0.11 hr at 70°C, 0.1 M solution). Many nonequilibrium reactions were described.	2
Reaction with nucleophiles	Propane sultone was highly reactive as a sulfoalkylating agent with alcohols, phenols, amines, thiols, carboxylic acid salts, amides, sulfonamides, and inorganic salts.	3
Reaction with nucleophiles	The reactions with nucleosides and with pyridine were studied in dimethylsulfoxide.	4
Reaction with trialkyl-aluminum	A patent describing the preparation of sulfonate detergents from sultones.	5
Reaction with aziridines	The ring of propane sultone opened as it polymerized with various aziridines.	6
Reaction with 4-(p-nitroben-zyl)-pyridine Hydrolysis	1,3-Propane sultone alkylated 4-(p-nitrobenzyl)-pyridine to give a colored product. Propane sultone was also hydrolyzed in aqueous solutions. These reactions were temperature dependent. Data with other sultones and cyclic sulfate esters were included.	7
Hydrolysis	$T_{1/2}$ in phosphate buffer, pH 7.4, at 37°C, was 110 min. Carcinogenicity and physical properties were studied. Included data for 1,4-butane sultone.	8
Hydrolysis	A kinetic study was made of the hydrolysis mechanism.	9
Solvolysis	A kinetic study was made of ring-opening in binary solvents containing water in varied proportions at three temperatures.	10

1,3-Propane Sultone

1. Osterman-Golkar, S. and Wachtmeister, C. A. On the reaction kinetics in water of 1,3-propane sultone and 1,4-butane sultone: A comparison of reaction rates and mutagenic activities of some alkylating agents. *Chem.-Biol. Interact.* **14**:195–202, 1976.
2. Fischer, R. F. Propanesultone. *Ind. Eng. Chem.* **56**(3):41–45, 1964.
3. Gilbert, E. E. Sulfonation and sulfation. In: *Kirk-Othmer Encyclopedia of Chemical Technology, 2nd. ed.* **19**:920. John Wiley & Sons, New York, 1969.
4. Goldschmidt, B. M., Frenkel, K., and Van Duuren, B. L. The reaction of propane sultone with guanosine, adenosine, and related compounds. *J. Heterocycl. Chem.* **11**:719–722, 1974.
5. Van Venrooy, J. J. Sulfonates from sultones. *U.S. Patent #4,012,400,* March 15, 1977.
6. Hashimoto, S., Yamashita, T., and Ono, M. Ring-opening polymerization of sultones. IX. Copolymerization of 3-hydroxy-1-propane sulfonic acid sultone and 1-substituted aziridines. *Kobunshi Ronbunshu* **33**:373–379, 1976.
7. Fischer, G. W., Jentzsch, R., Kasanzewa, V., and Riemer, F. Reactivity and toxicity of cyclic sulfuric acid esters. *J. Prakt. Chem.* **317**:943–952, 1975.
8. Druckrey, H., Kruse, H., Preussmann, R., Ivankovic, S., Landschütz, Ch., and Gimmy, J. Cancerogenic alkylating substances. IV. 1,3-Propane sultone and 1,4-butane sultone. *Z. Krebsforsch.* **75**:69–84, 1970.
9. Mori, A., Nagayama, M., and Mandai, H. Mechanism and reactivity of hydrolysis of aliphatic sulfonate esters. *Bull. Chem. Soc. Jpn.* **44**:1669–1672, 1971.
10. Massiff de la Fuente, G. Effect of solvent on the solvolysis of 1,3-propane sultone. *An. Fac. Quim. Farm. Univ. Chile* **21**:45–48, 1969.

CARBOXYLIC ACID DERIVATIVES

ETHIONINE
(67-21-0: D,L-ISOMER)
(13073-35-3: L-ISOMER)
(55-17-4: UNSPECIFIED ISOMER)

Degradation Technique	Remarks	Reference
Microbial	A strain of ethionine-resistant enteric yeast, *Candida slooffii*, degraded ethionine to unidentified substances.	1
Microbial	*E. coli* utilized ethionine as a sulfur source in the presence of NH_4 Cl.	2
Thermal	Decomposes at about 257–284°C.	3
Photo-decomposition	Ethylene was the main product formed when ethionine was irradiated with a fluorescent lamp in the presence of flavine mononucleotide. The reaction was pH dependent.	4

Ethionine

1. Mendonca, L. C. S. and Travassos, L. R. Metabolism of ethionine in eth-ionine-sensitive and ethionine-resistant cells of the enteric yeast *Candida slooffii. J. Bacteriol.* 110:643–651, 1972.
2. Faith, W. T. and Mallette, M. F. Biosynthesis of 3-ethylthiopropionic acid and degradation of ethionine by *Escherichia coli. Arch. Biochem. Biophys.* 117:75–83, 1966.
3. *The Merck Index, 9th ed.:* entry #3665, Windholz, M., Buavari, S., Stroumt-sos, L. Y., and Fertig, M. N. (Eds.). Merck and Co., Rahway, New Jersey, 1976.
4. Yang, S.-F. Photosensitized conversion of ethionine to ethylene by flavine monoucleotide. *Photochem. Photobiol.* 12:419–422, 1970.

β-PROPIOLACTONE (57-57-8)

Degradation Technique	Remarks	Reference
Hydrolysis	The kinetics was studied in acid, neutral, and basic solutions. Rate constants were determined for the different conditions.	1
Hydrolysis	67% was hydrolyzed at pH 7.4, 22–24°C, in 30 min. After 3 hr at 22–24°C and 48 hr at 4°C, 93% had hydrolyzed.	2
Hydrolysis	The rate was markedly affected by temperature, but the only value cited was a $T_{1/2}$ of 210 min at room temperature. No details.	3
Hydrolysis	In a 5% immunoglobulin IgG solution in 0.9% NaCl, pH 8, at 37°C, $T_{1/2}$ of BPL was 25 min.	4
Hydrolysis	A kinetic analysis of the hydrolysis of BPL catalyzed by imidazole at pH 6.3–8.6.	5
Hydrolysis Reaction with $Na_2 S_2 O_3$	The rate constant in hydrolysis was 11.3×10^{-3}/min at 37°C; in reaction with $Na_2 S_2 O_3$, it was 0.13 ℓ/mole/sec at 24°C.	6
Hydrolysis Reaction with cysteine	Rate constants were determined at 25°C. The product formed with cysteine had only very weak carcinogenicity.	7
Hydrolysis Reaction with $NH_2 OH$	$T_{1/2}$ was 210 min at 25°C, 5 min at 75°C. Reacted quantitatively with $NH_2 OH$ to give hydroxamic acid. Physical and chemical properties of BPL were included.	8
Hydrolysis Reaction with $NaNO_2$	In unbuffered solution, with an initial pH of 3.9, 50% was hydrolyzed in 4 hr at 20°C, and 94% in 1 hr at 60°C. Sodium 3-nitropropionate was formed at pH 7.5 and was used for the polargraphic analysis of BPL.	9
Hydrolysis Reaction with nucleophiles	$T_{1/2}$ of aqueous solutions was about 0.5–3 hr at 25°C. It was highly reactive with nucleophiles such as thiols. A review; no details.	10
Hydrolysis Reaction with nucleophiles	A review, including chemical aspects of BPL as a carcinogen.	11

β-PROPIOLACTONE (57–57–8)
(continued)

Degradation Technique	Remarks	Reference
Reaction with nucleophiles	A kinetic study was made of the reactions with several reagents. Degradation occurred most rapidly with $S_2O_3^=$ and OH^-, apparently by different mechanisms.	12
Reaction with cysteine	Cysteine and BPL reacted at pH 7, 20°C, for 2.5 hr, to give a high yield of addition product.	13
Reaction with amino acids	At pH's of 3, 7, or 9, methionine was usually most reactive.	14
Reaction with thioureas	Reaction with N-methyl isothiourea in water gave 91% N-methyl-S-(2-carboxyethyl)-isothiourea. Other reactions were described.	15
Chemical	A review of the properties and chemistry of BPL. Reactions with many chemical agents were cited.	16
Thermal	First order gas phase decomposition gave stoichiometric amounts of C_2H_4 and CO_2 at 205–255°C.	17
Thermal Oxidation	Boiling point was 162°C with decomposition. Flash point: 70°C.	18
Polymerization	Polymerization, when catalyzed by acids, bases, or salts, could be explosive. The polymer was degraded by alkali, reaction with alcohols at acid pH, or pyrolysis at 150°C.	19
	First aid and handling of spills are described.	20

BPL: β-propiolactone

β-Propiolactone

1. Long, F. A. and Purchase, M. The kinetics of hydrolysis of β-propiolactone in acid, neutral and basic solutions. *J. Am. Chem. Soc.* 72:3267–3273, 1950.
2. Schmitz-Masse, M. O. Gas-liquid chromatographic analysis of β-propiolactone. *J. Chromatogr.* 70:128–134, 1972.

3. Künzel, W. The possibilities of sterilization with beta-propiolactone. *Wiss. Z. Univ. Rostock Math. Naturwiss. Reihe* **19**:263–265, 1970.
4. Pruggmayer, D. and Stephan, W. Gas chromatographic trace analysis of β-propiolactone in sterilized serum proteins. *Vox Sang.* **31**:191–198, 1976.
5. Blackburn, G. M. and Duce, D. Strain effects in acyl transfer reactions. Part 4. Kinetic analysis of the reaction of imidazole buffer solutions with β-propiolactone using a novel graphical method for branched, series reactions. *J. Chem. Soc., Perkin Trans.* 2:1492–1498, 1977.
6. Van Duuren, B. L. and Goldschmidt, B. M. Carcinogenicity of epoxides, lactones, and peroxy compounds. III. Biological activity and chemical reactivity. *J. Med. Chem.* **9**:77–79, 1966.
7. Dickens, F. and Jones, H. E. H. Carcinogenic activity of a series of reactive lactones and related substances. *Br. J. Cancer* **15**:85–100, 1961.
8. Hoffman, R. K. and Warshowsky, B. *Beta*-Propiolactone vapor as a disinfectant. *Appl. Microbiol.* **6**:358–362, 1958.
9. Pellerin, F. and Letavernier, J.-F. Polarographic detection of β-propiolactone. *Ann. Pharm. Fr.* **32**:561–568, 1974.
10. Fishbein, L. Degradation and residues of alkylating agents. *Ann. N.Y. Acad. Sci.* **163**:878–880, 1969.
11. Dickens, F. Carcinogenic lactones and related substances. *Br. Med. Bull.* **20**:96–101, 1964.
12. Bartlett, P. D. and Small, G. Jr. β-Propiolactone. IX. The kinetics of attack by nucleophilic reagents upon the alcoholic carbon of β-propiolactone. *J. Am. Chem. Soc.* **72**:4867–4869, 1950.
13. Ichikawa, Y., Utsumi, S., and Kurisu, K. Studies on the antimicrobial action of propionate and related substances. Part I. The mechanism of the microbicidal action of β-propiolactone. *Nippon Nogai Kagaku Kaishi* **41**:84–93, 1967.
14. Taubman, M. A. and Atassi, M. Z. Reaction of β-propiolactone with amino acids and its specificity for methionine. *Biochem. J.* **106**:829–834, 1968.
15. Hanefeld, W. Studies of 1,3-thiazines. VI. Cyclization reactions of N-monosubstituted thioureas with 1,3-reactive propionyl derivatives. *Arch. Pharm. (Weinheim)* **310**:273–285, 1977.
16. Machell, G. Properties and reactions of *beta*-propiolactone. *Ind. Chem.* **36**:13–20, 1960.
17. James, T. L. and Wellington, C. A. Thermal decomposition of β-propiolactone in the gas phase. *J. Am. Chem. Soc.* **91**:7743–7746, 1969.
18. *The Merck Index, 9th ed.:* entry #7610, Windholz, M., Buavari, S., Stroumtsos, L. Y., and Fertig, M. N. (Eds.). Merck and Co., Rahway, New Jersey, 1976.
19. Gresham, T. L., Jansen, J. E., and Shaver, F. W. β-Propiolactone. I. Polymerization reactions. *J. Am. Chem. Soc.* **70**:998–1001, 1948.
20. *Hazards in the Chemical Laboratory, 2nd ed.:* 371, Muir, G. D. (Ed.). The Chemical Society, London, 1977.

URETHANE (51-79-6)

Degradation Technique	Remarks	Reference
Hydrolysis	Rate constants were determined for the alkaline hydrolysis of urethane and other carbamate esters at various temperatures and hydroxyl ion concentrations.	1
Hydrolysis	Unsubstituted esters of carbamic acid produced stoichiometric amounts of NH_3 when boiled in 4–5% NaOH in the presence of a Raney Ni catalyst containing 3–4% Al.	2
Hydrolysis	The rate of urethane decomposition by acids was studied at $37^\circ C$.	3
Hydrolysis	The decomposition of urethane by acids was further studied.	4

Urethane

1. Dittert, L. W. and Higuchi, T. Rates of hydrolysis of carbamate and carbonate esters in alkaline solution. *J. Pharm. Sci.* 52:852–857, 1963.
2. Tóth, Z. and Krasznai, I. A method for the determination of the esters of carbamic acid. *Magy. Kém. Foly.* 65:289–291, 1959.
3. Pedersen, K. J. The rate of decomposition of urethane in acid solution. *Acta Chem. Scand.* 14:1448–1449, 1960.
4. Pedersen, K. J. The rate of decomposition of urethane in acid solution II. *Acta Chem. Scand.* 15:959, 1961.

AZO AND AZOXY DERIVATIVES

DIAZOMETHANE (334-88-3)

Degradation Technique	Remarks	Reference
Physico-chemical	Undiluted liquid or concentrated solutions may explode if impurities, solids, or rough surfaces (e.g., ground glass) are present. Even when diluted with N_2, it may explode at $100^\circ C$ or above, or under high-intensity light.	1
Physico-chemical	Hazardous reactions cited. First aid mentioned.	2
Physico-chemical Polymerization Reaction with nucleophiles	May explode at $100^\circ C$, or in contact with ground glass surfaces or alkali metals. In the presence of Cu, insoluble polymethylene and N_2 formed. Diazomethane methylated thio, acidic hydroxyl, amino, and imino groups. No details	3
Polymerization	Polymethylene was produced in the dark in the presence of carbon black.	4
Polymerization	Polymethylene was produced by the catalytic acid of tetrakis (phenyldiethoxyphosphine) cobalt hydride in ether.	5
Reaction with nucleophiles	The rate increased with the acidity of the proton donor. Phenols formed aryl methyl ethers. Alcohols could be etherified when HBF_4 was added to the system as proton donor.	6
Reaction with guanosine	Variations of products were studied under varied conditions of reaction.	7
Hydrolysis	The kinetics of the perchloric acid-catalyzed hydrolysis of dilute diazomethane were studied by slowing the reaction with tetrahydrofuran.	8
Photo-decomposition	Diazomethane in ether did not react with water unless exposed to sunlight. CH_3OH and N_2 were formed.	9

DIAZOMETHANE (334-88-3)
(continued)

Degradation Technique	Remarks	Reference
Photo-decomposition	An ethereal solution of diazomethane was decomposed by sunlight to form N_2, C_2H_4, a slight amount of $(CH_2)_x$, and methylated derivatives of ether.	10
Photo-decomposition	A kinetic study of photolysis with NH_3 and with CH_3NH_2.	11
Photo-decomposition	A kinetic study of the photolysis of diazomethane in methanol and in ethanol. Products were identified.	12

Diazomethane

1. *Handbook of Reactive Chemical Hazards:* 234, Bretherick, L. (Ed.). CRC Press, Cleveland, Ohio, 1975.
2. *Hazards in the Chemical Laboratory, 2nd ed.:* 214, Muir, G. D. (Ed.). The Chemical Society, London, 1977.
3. *Int. Agency Res. Cancer Monogr.* 7:223, Lyon, France, 1974.
4. Wicker-Coudurier, G., Shingal, R., and Donnet, J. B. Diazomethane decomposition in the presence of carbon black. *Bull. Soc. Chim. Fr.:* 1704–1711, 1970.
5. Mazzi, U., Orio, A. A., Nicolini, M., and Marzotto, A. Catalytic decomposition of diazomethane to polymethylene. *Atti Accad. Peloritana Pericolanti, Cl. Sci. Fis. Mat. Natur.* 50:95–98, 1970.
6. Gutsche, C. D. and Pasto, D. J. *Fundamentals of Organic Chemistry:* 693–694. Prentice-Hall, Englewood Cliffs, New Jersey, 1975.
7. Sullivan, J. P. and Wong, J. L. Guanosine-methyldiazonium ion reaction: variation of methylation product patterns with reaction variables. *Biochem. Biophys. Acta* 479:1–15, 1977.
8. McGarrity, J. F. and Smyth, T. Kinetics and mechanism of the acid-catalyzed hydrolysis of diazomethane. *J. Chem. Soc., Chem. Commun.:* 347–348, 1977.
9. Palazzo, F. C. An interesting aspect of the behavior of diazomethane. *Gazz. Chim. Ital.* 79:13–24, 1949.
10. Meerwein, H., Rathjen, H., and Werner, H. Methylation of RH compounds by diazomethane under the action of light. *Ber. Dtsch. Chem. Ges. B* 75: 1610–1622, 1942.

11. Ho, S.-Y. and Tong, S.-N. Photochemistry of diazomethane. Reaction of methylene with ammonia and methylamine. *J. Chin. Chem. Soc. (Taipei)* **19**:189–195, 1972.
12. Ho, S.-Y. and Lin, H.-B. Photochemistry of diazomethane. Reactions of methylene with methanol and ethanol. *J. Chin. Chem. Soc. (Taipei)* **20**: 27–33, 1973.

CYCASIN (14901-08-7)

Degradation Technique	Remarks	Reference
Hydrolysis	Destroyed by treatment with alkali.	1
Hydrolysis	Methylazoxymethanol (aglycone of cycasin) decomposed at $37°C$ in D_2O: $T_{1/2}$ was 18.6 hr. HCHO, methanol and N_2 were products.	2
Hydrolysis	Easily hydrolyzed, especially at alkaline pH, to yield N_2, HCHO, methanol and other products. No details.	3
Hydrolysis Reduction Thermal	1 N HCl produced N_2, HCHO, and methanol. Reduction with $SnCl_2$ and HCl gave glucose, CH_3NH_2, NH_3, and HCHO. Cycasin melted at $144-145°C$, with decomposition.	4
Hydrolysis Thermal	1 N HCl at $97°C$ produced D-glucose, HCHO, and N_2. Cycasin melted at $154°C$, with decomposition.	5
Hydrolysis Thermal	A 10^{-3} M aqueous solution of methylazoxymethanol was decomposed 75% in 30 min at $75°C$, and 100% in 10 min at $100°C$. Esters yielded HCHO quantitatively when hydrolyzed with acid. HCHO was released quantitatively when methylazoxymethanol was heated (no details). About 11% was decomposed in five days at $30°C$.	6
	Cysteamine protected mice from the lethality of the aglycone (methylazoxymethanol) *in vivo*.	7

Cycasin

1. Kobayashi, A., Yamauchi, H., and Murozono, T. Analysis of the residual cycasin in food products made from cycad. *Kagoshima Diagaku Nogakubu Gakujutsu Hokoku* 24:165–170, 1974.
2. Nagasawa, H. T., Shirota, F. N., and Matsumoto, H. Decomposition of methylazoxymethanol, the aglycone of cycasin, in D_2O. *Nature* 236:234–235, 1972.
3. *Int. Agency Res. Cancer Monogr.* 10:121, Lyon, France, 1976.
4. Nishida, K., Kobayashi, A., and Nagahama, T. Cycasin, a toxic glycoside of *Cycas revoluta*. I. Isolation and structure of cycasin. *Bull. Agric. Chem. Soc. Jpn.* 19:77–84, 1955.
5. Riggs, N. V. Glucosyloxyazoxymethane, a constitutent of the seeds of *Cycas circinalis* L. *Chem. Ind. (London):* 926, 1956.
6. Kobayashi, A. and Matsumoto, H. Studies on methylazoxymethanol, the aglycone of cycasin. Isolation, biological, and chemical properties. *Arch. Biochem. Biophys.* 110:373–380, 1965.
7. Miwa, T. Studies on the protective effect of radioprotective compounds against the hepatotoxic and carcinogenic activity of methylazoxymethanol. *Acta Sch. Med. Univ. Gifu* 23:495–500, 1975.

o-AMINOAZOTOLUENE (97-56-3)

Degradation Technique	Remarks	Reference
Reduction	Zn dust + HCl→toulene-2,5-diamine. No details.	1
Reaction with dialkyl acetylenedicarboxylates	The addition of dialkyl acetylenedicarboxylates to carcinogenic amines was described. *o*-Aminoazotoluene gave 87% yield of product, which was to be tested for carcinogenicity.	2

o-Aminoazoltoluene

1. Thirtle, J. R. Phenylenediamines and toluenediamines. In: *Kirk-Othmer Encyclopedia of Chemical Technology, 2nd ed.* 15:217. John Wiley & Sons, New York, 1968.
2. Iwanami, Y. The reaction of acetylenecarboxylic acid with amines. XVII. The addition of dialkyl acetylenedicarboxylates to several carcinogens. *Bull. Chem. Soc. Jpn.* 48:1657–1658, 1975.

p-DIMETHYLAMINOAZOBENZENE (60-11-7)

Degradation Technique	Remarks	Reference
Photo-decomposition	The relative stabilities of DMAB and its derivatives to UV radiation were determined in various solvents.	1
Oxidation	A study of the oxidation by $Ce(SO_4)_2$ in acid at $20°C$. A number of products were identified.	2

DMAB: p-dimethylaminoazobenzene

p-Dimethylaminoazobenzene

1. Rambousek, V., Sagner, Z., Matrka, M., and Marhold, J. Oxidation of carcinogenic azo dyes. XI. Decomposition of N,N-dimethyl-4-aminoazobenzene and its metabolites by light during isolation and determination. *Collect. Czech. Chem. Commun.* 35:3784–3788, 1970.
2. Matrka, M. and Marhold, J. Oxidation of carcinogenic azo dyes. II. Oxidation of N,N-dimethyl-4-aminoazobenzene by cerium (IV) sulfate. *Collect. Czech. Chem. Commun.* 33:4273–4282, 1968.

3'-METHYL-4-AMINOAZOBENZENE (722-23-6)

Degradation Technique	Remarks	Reference
Reaction with dialkyl acetylenedicarboxylates	The addition of dialkyl acetylenedicarboxylates to carcinogenic amines was described. This primary amine was not included, but probably would react in a similar manner.	1

3'-Methyl-4-aminoazobenzene

1. Iwanami, Y. The reaction of acetylenecarboxylic acid with amines. XVII. The addition of dialkyl acetylenedicarboxylates to several carcinogens. *Bull. Chem. Soc. Jpn.* 48:1657–1658, 1975.

AFLATOXINS

AFLATOXINS*
(B_1: 1162–65–8)
(B_2: 7220–81–7)
(G_1: 1165–39–5)

Degradation Technique	Remarks	Reference
Oxidation	UV lamp used to monitor fluorescence of nondegraded residues after treatment of work surfaces, skin, mouth, clothing, glassware, etc., with solutions of various oxidizing agents.	1
Oxidation	A 1:9 dilution of 5–6% NaOCl (Clorox) provided safe cleanup of glassware and work surfaces when used thoroughly.	2
Oxidation	Effects of concentration, pH, temperature, and time were studied. 0.3% NaOCl, pH 9–10, for 30 min, effectively destroyed B_1 and B_2 in the protein isolates from peanuts.	3
Oxidation	B_1 toxicity was destroyed by treatment with H_2O_2 for 0.5 hr at 80°C, pH 9.5. Tests were made with pure B_1 as well as with contaminated peanut meal.	4
Oxidation	Peanut meal was detoxified by treatment with H_2O_2 in an alkaline medium for 20 min at 70°C.	5
Oxidation	The probable oxidation products were considered in detail after treatment of B_1 with m-chloroperoxybenzoic acid.	6
Oxidation Reduction	Oxidation of B_1 with H_2O_2 in NaOH produced succinic acid as one product. Reduction produced the dihydro derivative (B_2) or tetrahydrodesoxo-B_1, depending upon conditions.	7
Reduction	The already degraded B_{2a} molecule was reduced by $NaBH_4$. Neither product was toxic to chick embryos at levels 100 times the LD_{50} of B_1.	8

*In this section, B_1, B_2, G_1, etc., refer to the various structural forms of aflatoxins.

AFLATOXINS
(continued)

Degradation Technique	Remarks	Reference
Hydroxylation	Treatment of B_1 with 0.1 N citric acid for 1–2 days at $28°C$ produced hydroxydihydroaflatoxin B_1 (B_{2a}) which was less toxic than the parent B_1.	9
Hydroxylation	Water addition occurred during treatment with 1N H_2SO_4 for 10 min at $70°C$ to form B_{2a}, the hemiacetal.	10
Hydroxylation	Conditions were determined for the production of about 90% hemiacetal of B_1 in acid solution. The hemiacetal (B_{2a}) was biologically inactive in chick embryo and *in vitro* lung cell tests.	11
Hydroxylation	Treatment of B_1 and G_1 with cold, dilute, aqueous, mineral acid caused the addition of water to form B_{2a} and G_{2a}, which were much less toxic than the parent compounds. No details of acid treatment.	12
Hydroxylation	A kinetic study of the rates of conversion of B_1 and G_1 to less toxic hemiacetals, B_{2a} and G_{2a}, in dilute H_2SO_4. At pH 1, 95% conversion of B_1 occurred in 10 min at $100°C$, and in 3 hr at $40°C$.	13
Ozonation	Treatment of moist oilseed meals with O_3 at $100°C$ was effective in destroying B_1 and G_1, but not B_2, as indicated by TLC analysis. The effects of moisture, time, and temperature were studied.	14
Ozonation	Treatment with O_3 for 1–2 hr at $75–100°C$ in the presence of moisture lowered the B_1 content of oilseed meals from 82 ppb to 18 ppb.	15
Photo-decomposition	B_1 and G_1 were unstable in aqueous solution in daylight: 40% decomposition/day; almost 100%/nine days.	16
Photo-decomposition	Exposure of B_1 to UV radiation on TLC plate resulted in a degradation product.	17

AFLATOXINS
(continued)

Degradation Technique	Remarks	Reference
Photo-decomposition	Degradation of B_1 by UV radiation was affected by the solvent used and by the presence of riboflavin, KI, and ascorbic acid.	18
Photo-decomposition	Photoproducts of B_1 formed much faster on silica gel plates than in methanol solution. The principal product was less toxic than B_1. The product was converted to nonfluorescent substances by strong acids.	19
Photo-decomposition	Products containing solvent adducts were isolated after UV irradiation of aflatoxins in ethanol or methanol. The products were less toxic for chicken embryos than were the parent compounds.	20
Photo-decomposition	UV irradiation of B_1 in chloroform reduced its toxicity in 1–2 hr. Oilseed meals might be treated as a thin layer on a conveyor belt.	21
Photo-decomposition Hydrolysis	Exposure of B_1 or G_1 to UV reduced its toxicity for chick embryos, possibly by eliminating the furan double bond or the furan ring itself. NaOH opened the lactone ring and allowed reaction with p-nitrobenzenediazonium fluoroborate to give a brick-red product.	22
Photo-decomposition Ionizing radiation Thermal	The kinetics of changes in the physicochemical and biological properties of B_1 during radiation were studied. Melting point data indicated that pure aflatoxins melt between $237°$ and $299°C$ with decomposition.	23
Ionizing radiation	Studies were made, using an electron beam. Dry aflatoxins required such large doses of radiation that the foods were adversely affected. Aflatoxins in aqueous solutions were much more easily destroyed by the radiation.	24
Ammoniation	Treatment of B_1 with NH_4OH for 0.5–8 hr at $100°C$ in a Parr bomb gave products devoid of the lactone ring, with or without the cyclopentanone ring.	25

AFLATOXINS
(continued)

Degradation Technique	Remarks	Reference
Ammoniation	Time, temperature, and pressure effects were studied for detoxifying peanut meal. Abstract only; no details.	26
Ammoniation	Destruction of aflatoxin with NH_3 had no effect on egg laying of hens fed treated cottonseed meal. Loss of cystine was compensated for by supplementing the diet with sulfur-containing amino acids.	27
Ammoniation	Conditions for the destruction of aflatoxins in agricultural products were described. Best results were obtained with 10–15% water + NH_3 at 200–250°F in an autoclave.	28
Ammoniation	Optimum conditions (NH_3, pressure, temperature, moisture content, time) were determined for the destruction of aflatoxins in cottonseed and peanut meals.	29
Ammoniation	The difuran rings of B_1 were implicated in the irreversible reaction with the protein and water-soluble fractions of corn rather than the starch. A marked reduction or complete loss of toxicity occurred in the chick embryo test after ammoniation if the contamination with B_1 did not exceed 27 mg/kg.	30
Ammoniation	Reaction of B_1 with 5 N NH_4OH for 18 days at ambient temperature resulted in about 50% conversion to products nontoxic to chick embryos.	31
Ammoniation	Studies with coumarin indicated that ammoniation under mild conditions may lead to β-amino derivatives when B_1 is similarly treated. No data with B_1.	32
Ammoniation	Treatment of moist corn with 1.5% NH_3 for 6–12 days at 49°C reduced aflatoxins from 180 ppb to nondetectable levels. Treatment markedly lowered the incidence of hepatomas in trout-feeding tests.	33

AFLATOXINS
(continued)

Degradation Technique	Remarks	Reference
Ammoniation	Greater than 99% detoxification was obtained when peanut meal was stored with 5% NH_3 and 20% water for ten days in plastic bags.	34
Ammoniation	Heating moist cottonseed meal with NH_3 under pressure at 200°F detoxified B_1 to form aflatoxin D_1, the ketoacid, and a product from which both the lactone and cyclopentanone rings were removed. Structures of 14 aflatoxins are given.	35
Ammoniation	Heating with NH_4OH at 100°C for 1 hr in a Parr bomb opened the lactone ring and released CO_2 from B_1. Similar results were obtained with 4% NaOH, but with lower yield of the main product, D_1.	36
Reaction with ammonia or methylamine	Treatment for 30 min at 93–100°C markedly lowered the aflatoxin content of cottonseed meal.	37
Reaction with methylamine	Dry or moist (preferred) treatment at 75–100°C with elimination of excess methylamine permitted use of contaminated products for animal feeds.	38
Hydrolysis	A study of the products obtained from B_1 during treatment with NaOH or diethanolamine at 20°C and at 100°C. Toxicity of the products was discussed.	39
Hydrolysis, washing, bleaching	Commercial refining procedures eliminated toxic aflatoxins from vegetable oils. Alkaline hydrolysis of the lactone ring eliminated fluorescence but not toxicity, since the ring readily closed again on acidification.	40
Hydrolysis Oxidation	Reactions of aflatoxins with many reagents were discussed. Degradation and detoxification were based on loss of fluorescence, changes in TLC R_f values, as well as chick embryo and	41

AFLATOXINS
(continued)

Degradation Technique	Remarks	Reference
	tissue culture bioassays. The need for more definitive animal toxicity studies was mentioned.	
Chemical	^{14}C-labeled B_1 was degraded by various organic reactions to locate positions of 13 of the 17 C-atoms.	42
Chemical	Various degradation procedures were used for determining the sources of 13 of the 17 C-atoms of B_1.	43
Chemical	A review, with 37 references, considering oxidizing agents, acids, and bases as means for detoxifying aflatoxins in foods and feeds.	44
Chemical	Evaluated various treatments for decontaminating oilseed meals, using reagents such as NH_3, $CH_3 NH_2$, $NaOH$, and $HCHO$.	45
Chemical	Treatment of moist peanut meal at elevated temperatures with NH_3, $CH_3 NH_2$, $NaOH$, or O_3 destroyed or greatly reduced aflatoxins, as indicated by TLC analysis and feeding tests with ducklings and rats.	46
Chemical	Among chemicals tested, $H_2 O_2$, $NaOCl$, and benzoyl peroxide were very effective for destroying aflatoxins during an aqueous extraction process for peanuts.	47
Chemical	The aflatoxin content of peanut meal was effectively lowered by the addition of 1–5%, by weight, of $NH_4 OH$, urea, $NH_4 HCO_3$, NH_4 isobutyrate, NH_4 propionate, or NH_4 acetate.	48
Chemical	Treatment with $Ca(OH)_2$, alone or with $HCHO$, in the presence of moisture, caused a marked decrease of aflatoxins in peanut meal.	49

AFLATOXINS
(continued)

Degradation Technique	Remarks	Reference
Microbial Chemical	About 1000 different microorganisms were tested. A *Flavobacterium* species was able to destroy B_1 and G_1 alone or in foods, without producing toxic products. Incubation for four days at $28°C$, pH 9.5, destroyed 50% of B_1 without bacteria, but the toxicity of the products was not tested.	50
Physico- chemical Microbial	A review, with 78 references, containing small sections on the general principles of detoxification of foods. No details.	51
Microbial	Various microorganisms degraded B_1, but some of the products were only slightly modified from the parent compounds. Degradation by some molds was almost complete in 20 days.	52
Microbial	*Aspergillus flavus* produced aflatoxin, but also degraded up to 55% in a few days under conditions of mycelial lysis and high aeration.	53
Microbial	75% of B_1 was degraded by starved cells of *Tetrahymena pyriformis* in 30 hr at $25°C$. G_1 was not degraded.	54
Microbial	A strain of *Norcardia asteroides* rapidly converted a crude B_1 preparation to non-fluorescent material. Purified B_1 was more resistant to degradation.	55
Microbial	B_1 formed a compound 18 times less toxic after incubation with *Dactylium dendroides*.	56
Microbial	*Rhizopus* species degraded about 60% of B_1 to isomeric hydroxy derivatives of the cyclopentanone ring during incubation for one week at $27°C$.	57
Microbial	G_1 was completely degraded after four weeks of incubation with a *Rhizopus* species at $27°C$. The terminal lactone group of G_1 was absent from the monolactone product (B_3 or parasiticol).	58

AFLATOXINS
(continued)

Degradation Technique	Remarks	Reference
Microbial	Incubation for ten days at 25°C with *Aspergillus candidus* partially degraded B_1 to an unidentified product ten times less toxic than B_1 for chick embryos.	59
Microbial	A *Dactylium dendroides* strain reduced the carbonyl group on the cyclopentane ring of B_1 to form aflatoxicol, which was 18 times less toxic than the parent compound.	60
Microbial	Several fungi (especially *Dactylium dendroides*) transformed 50–60% of B_1 into a hydroxylated derivative (aflatoxicol).	61
Microbial	Aflatoxins were degraded by 8- and 16-day-old mycelia of *Aspergillus parasiticus*.	62
Microbial	B_1 was degraded by only 3 of 18 microorganisms tested.	63
Microbial	Greater than 60% of aflatoxins were lost during the fermentation of grains. Further processing of the protein concentrate eliminated more than 90% of the toxins.	64
Microbial	B_1 was degraded by several microorganisms. Among the products was aflatoxin R_o (or aflatoxicol, in which the cyclopentanone group of B_1 is reduced to an hydroxyl group).	65
Thermal	120°C (15 psi) for 4 hr destroyed most of the B_1 in moist peanut meal. Pure B_1 or G_1 appeared to be completely destroyed by the same treatment.	66
Thermal	About 1.5–2% of B_1 was decomposed per hr when refluxed in methanol.	67
Thermal	Aflatoxin M_1 was stable in milk during pasteurization and subsequent storage for up to 17 days at 4°C. Only 45% was lost during frozen storage for 120 days at –18°C.	68

AFLATOXINS
(continued)

Degradation Technique	Remarks	Reference
Thermal	About 80% of B_1 plus B_2 was destroyed in cottonseed meal in 2 hr at $100°C$ with 20% moisture at atmospheric pressure. Only 34% was destroyed in peanut meal under these conditions.	69
Thermal	No destruction of aflatoxins in cooking oils occurred at less than $250°C$. Thus, little detoxification would occur during normal frying.	70
Thermal Oxidation	5% NaOCl solution was used for the disposal of aflatoxin-contaminated materials and for decontamination of hood surfaces; 10% chlorine gas decontaminated peanut meal overnight. Aflatoxins are decomposed at temperatures of $300°C$ or above.	71
Microbial Thermal Chemical	A review of many procedures tested with food products (peanuts, peanut meal, cottonseed meal, etc.).	72
Microbial Thermal Chemical	Includes a review of various methods proposed for the detoxification of peanut and cottonseed meals.	73
Microbial Thermal Chemical	A review, with 230 references, covering toxicity, production by various molds, analysis, and detoxification.	74
Microbial Thermal Chemical	A review, with 74 references, covering toxicity, occurrence in foods, analysis, and detoxification of foods.	75
Microbial Thermal Oxidation Ammoniation	A review, discussing methods for preventing, removing, and destroying aflatoxin contamination in foods and feeds. No details; 46 references.	76
Photodecomposition Hydrolysis Thermal Oxidation	Unstable to light and air, especially in highly polar solvents (stable for years in $CHCl_3$ in dark, cold). Lactone ring is susceptible to alkaline hydrolysis; totally destroyed by autoclaving in the presence of NH_3; destroyed by	77

AFLATOXINS
(continued)

Degradation Technique	Remarks	Reference
	hypochlorite; partly destroyed by cooking. No details.	
Hydroxylation Reduction Ozonation Thermal Photo- decomposition	A review article, giving few details (71 refer- ences). Partial decomposition, upon standing in methanolic solution, was accelerated by light or heat.	78
Reaction with ethylene oxide and/or methyl formate	About 95% of B_1 was destroyed by the treat- ment of peanuts for 16 hr with 1.5 g/ℓ of a 1:1 mixture of the gases at a moisture content of 16%.	79
Microbial Chemical Thermal	A review article, with few details (35 references). The removal or degradation of aflatoxins in foods and feeds is discussed, along with methods for preventing contamination.	80
Hydrolysis of dihalides Oxidation	The dichloride and dibromide of B_1 were pre- pared and hydrolyzed at pH 7.4, 21°C. $T_{1/2}$ was 30 sec for the dibromide, 180 sec for the dichloride. B_1 was oxidized with m-chloroper- benzoic acid to give $trans$-glycol derivatives.	81
Hydrolysis of dichloride	B_1 dichloride was prepared. $T_{1/2}$ for hydrolysis in 10% dimethylsulfoxide at pH 7.4, 37°C, was 0.5 min. The dichloride was highly carcino- genic and mutagenic, but the hydrolysis products were inactive under the test conditions.	82
Ammoniation	Treatment of peanut meal with gaseous NH_3 at 2–3 bars pressure destroyed up to 95% of the aflatoxins. Side effects seemed to be favorable for the use of treated meals by rumi- nants. Partial destruction of cystine may be compensated by the addition of methionine.	83
Microbial	Mycelia of *Aspergillus parasiticus* degraded B_1 and G_1. Fragmenting the mycelia greatly in- creased their ability to degrade aflatoxins.	84

AFLATOXINS
(continued)

Degradation Technique	Remarks	Reference
Microbial	Disrupted mycelia of nine-day-old *A. parasiticus* degraded G_1 approximately 1.6 times more rapidly than B_1. Degradation rates were approximately proportional to the concentrations of mycelia and aflatoxins.	85

Aflatoxins

1. Stoloff, L. and Trager, W. Recommended decontamination procedures for aflatoxin. *J. Assoc. Off. Agric. Chem.* 48:681–682, 1965.
2. Yang, C. Y. Comparative studies on the detoxification of aflatoxins by sodium hypochlorite and commercial bleaches. *Microbiol.* 24:885–890, 1972.
3. Natarajan, K. R., Rhee, K. C., Cater, C. M., and Mattil, K. F. Destruction of aflatoxins in peanut protein isolates by sodium hypochlorite. *J. Am. Oil Chem. Soc.* 52:160–163, 1975.
4. Spreenivasamurthy, V., Parpia, H. A. B., Srikanta, S., and Shankarmurti, A. Detoxification of aflatoxin in peanut meal by hydrogen peroxide. *J. Assoc. Off. Anal. Chem.* 50:350–354, 1967.
5. Parpia, H. A. B. and Sreenivasamurthy, V. Importance of aflatoxin in foods with reference to India. *Proc. Int. Congr. Food Sci. Technol., 3rd, 1970:* 701–704. Inst. Food Technol., Chicago, Illinois, 1971.
6. Lhoest, G., Dumont, P., Mercier, M., and Roberfroid, M. Oxidation routes of aflatoxin B_1. *Pharm. Acta Helv.* 50:145–150, 1975.
7. Van Dorp, D. A., Van Der Zijden, A. S. M., Beerthuis, R. K., Sparreboom, S., Ord, W. O., De Jong, K., and Keuning, R. Dihydro-aflatoxin B, a metabolite of *Asperigillus flavus*. Remarks on the structure of aflatoxin B. *Recl. Trav. Chim. Pays-Bas* 82:587–592, 1963.
8. Ashoor, S. H. and Chu, F. S. Reduction of aflatoxin B_{2a} with sodium borohydride. *J. Agric. Food Chem.* 23:445–447, 1975.
9. Ciegler, A. and Peterson, R. E. Aflatoxin detoxification: hydroxydihydroaflatoxin B_1. *Appl. Microbiol.* 16:665–666, 1968.
10. Scoppa, P. and Marafante, E. Fluorimetric determination of aflatoxin B_1 in aqueous solutions. *Ann. Microbiol. Enzimol.* 21:89–95, 1971.
11. Pohland, A. E., Cushmac, M. E., and Andrellos, P. J. Aflatoxin B_1 hemiacetal. *J. Assoc. Off. Anal. Chem.* 51:907–910, 1968.

12. Dutton, M. F. and Heathcote, J. G. The structure, biochemical properties and origin of the aflatoxins B_{2a} and G_{2a}. *Chem. Ind. (London):* 418–421, 1968.

13. Pons, W. A. Jr., Cucullu, A. F., Lee, L. S., Janssen, H. J., and Goldblatt, L. A. Kinetic study of acid-catalyzed conversion of aflatoxins B_1 and G_1 to B_{2a} and G_{2a}. *J. Am. Oil Chem. Soc.* 49:124–128, 1972.

14. Dwarakanath, C. T., Rayner, E. T., Mann, G. E., and Dollear, F. G. Reduction of aflatoxin levels in cottonseed and peanut meal by ozonization. *J. Am. Oil Chem. Soc.* 45:93–95, 1968.

15. Rayner, E. T., Dwarakanath, C. T., Channasamudram, T., Mann, G. E., and Dollear, F. G. Reduction of the aflatoxin content of oilseed meals by ozonization, *U.S. Patent #3,592,641,* July 13, 1971.

16. Lijinsky, W. and Butler, W. H. Purification and toxicity of aflatoxin G_1. *Proc. Soc. Exp. Biol. Med.* 123:151–154, 1966.

17. Shantha, T., Murthy, V. S., and Parpia, H. A. B. An integrated distinguishing test for aflatoxin. *J. Food Sci. Technol.* 11:194–196, 1974.

18. Joseph-Bravo, P. I., Findley, M., and Newberne, P. M. Some interactions of light, riboflavin, and aflatoxin B_1 *in vivo* and *in vitro. J. Toxicol. Environ. Health* 1:353–376, 1976.

19. Andrellos, P. J., Beckwith, A. C., and Eppley, R. M. Photochemical changes of aflatoxin B_1. *J. Assoc. Off. Anal. Chem.* 50:346–350, 1967.

20. Wei, R.-D. and Chu, F. S. Aflatoxin-solvent interactions induced by ultraviolet light. *J. Assoc. Off. Anal. Chem.* 56:1425–1430, 1973.

21. Arthur, J. C. Jr. and Robertson, J. A. Jr. Detoxification of aflatoxin. *U.S. Patent #3,506,452,* April 14, 1970.

22. Lillard, D. A. and Lantin, R. S. Some chemical characteristics and biological effects of photomodified aflatoxins. *J. Assoc. Off. Anal. Chem.* 53:1060–1063, 1970.

23. Aibara, K. and Miyaki, K. Aflatoxin and its radiosensitivity. In: *Radiation Sensitivity of Toxins and Animal Poisons:* 41–62. IAEA **PL-334/7**, Vienna, 1970.

24. Frank, H. K. and Grunewald, T. *Radiation Resistance of Aflatoxins.* IAEA Rep. **R-551-F**, Vienna, 1970.

25. Cucullu, A. F., Lee, L. S., Pons, W. A. Jr., and Stanley, J. B. Ammoniation of aflatoxin B_1: isolation and characterization of a product with molecular weight 206. *J. Agric. Food Chem.* 24:408–410, 1976.

26. Koltun, S. P., Rayner, E. T., and Tallant, J. D. Inactivation of aflatoxins in contaminated peanut meal by ammoniation on a pilot plant scale. *J. Am. Oil Chem. Soc.* 51:285A, 1974.

27. Waldroup, P. W., Hazen, K. R., Mitchell, R. J., Payne, J. R., and Johnson, Z. Ammoniated cottonseed meal as a protein supplement for laying hens. *Poult. Sci.* 55:1011–1019, 1976.

28. Masri, M. S., Vix, H. L. E., and Goldblatt, L. A. Process for detoxifying substances contaminated with aflatoxin. *U.S. Patent #3,429,709,* Feb. 25, 1969.
29. Gardner, H. K. Jr., Koltun, S. P., Dollear, F. G., and Rayner, E. T. Inactivation of aflatoxins in peanut and cottonseed meals by ammoniation. *J. Am. Oil Chem. Soc.* 48:70–73, 1971.
30. Beckwith, A. C., Vesonder, R. F., and Ciegler, A. Action of weak bases upon aflatoxin B_1 in contact with macromolecular reactants. *J. Agric. Food Chem.* 23:582–587, 1975.
31. Vesonder, R. F., Beckwith, A. C., Ciegler, A., and Dimler, R. J. Ammonium hydroxide treatment of aflatoxin B_1. Some chemical characteristics and biological effects. *J. Agric. Food Chem.* 23:242–243, 1975.
32. Bergot, B. J., Stanley, W. L., and Masri, M. S. Reaction of coumarin with aqua ammonia. Implications in detoxification of aflatoxin. *J. Agric. Food Chem.* 25:965–966, 1977.
33. Brekke, O. L., Sinnhuber, R. O., Peplinski, A. J., Wales, J. H., Putnam, G. B., Lee, D. J., and Ciegler, A. Aflatoxin in corn: ammonia inactivation and bioassay with rainbow trout. *Appl. Environ. Microbiol.* 34:34–37, 1977.
34. Thiesen, J. Detoxification of aflatoxins in groundnut meal. *Anim. Feed Sci. Technol.* 2:67–75, 1977.
35. Goldblatt, L. A. Mycotoxins—past, present and future. . . . *J. Am. Oil Chem. Soc.* 54:302A–309A, 1977.
36. Lee, L. S., Stanley, J. B., Cucullu, A. F., Pons, W. A. Jr., and Goldblatt, L. A. Ammoniation of aflatoxin B_1: isolation and identification of the major reaction product. *J. Assoc. Off. Anal. Chem.* 57:626–631, 1974.
37. Mann, G. E., Gardner, H. K. Jr., Booth, A. N., and Gumbmann, M. R. Aflatoxin inactivation. Chemical and biological properties of ammonia and methylamine treated cottonseed meal. *J. Agric. Food Chem.* 19:1155–1158, 1971.
38. Mann, G. E., Codifer, L. P. Jr., Gardner, H. K. Jr., and Dollear, F. G. Process for lowering aflatoxin levels in aflatoxin-contaminated substances. *U.S. Patent #3,585,041,* June 15, 1971.
39. Kiermeier, F. and Ruffer, L. Changes of aflatoxin B_1 in alkaline solutions. *Z. Lebensm. Unters.-Forsch.* 155:129–141, 1974.
40. Parker, W. A. and Melnick, D. Absence of aflatoxin from refined vegetable oils. *J. Am. Oil Chem. Soc.* 43:635–638, 1966.
41. Trager, W. and Stoloff, L. Possible reactions for aflatoxin detoxification. *J. Agric. Food Chem.* 15:679–681, 1967.
42. Biollaz, M., Buchi, G., and Milne, G. Biosynthesis of aflatoxins. *J. Am. Chem. Soc.* 90:5017–5019, 1968.
43. Biollaz, M., Buchi, G., and Milne, G. The biosynthesis of the aflatoxins. *J. Am. Chem. Soc.* 92:1035–1043, 1970.

44. Beckwith, A. C., Vesonder, R. F., and Ciegler, A. Chemical methods investigated for detoxifying aflatoxins in foods and feeds. In: *Mycotoxins and Other Fungal Related Food Problems:* 58–67, Rodricks, J. V. (Ed.). Adv. Chem. Ser. **149**, Am. Chem. Soc., Washington, D.C., 1976.
45. Mann, G. E., Codifer, L. P. Jr., Gardner, H. K. Jr., Koltun, S. P., and Dollear, F. G. Chemical inactivation of aflatoxins in peanut and cottonseed meals. *J. Am. Oil Chem. Soc.* **47**:173–176, 1970.
46. Dollear, F. G., Mann, G. E., Codifer, L. P. Jr., Gardner, H. K. Jr., Koltun, S. P., and Vix, H. L. E. Elimination of aflatoxins from peanut meal. *J. Am. Oil Chem. Soc.* **45**:862–865, 1968.
47. Rhee, K. C., Natarajan, K. R., Cater, C. M., and Mattil, K. F. Processing edible peanut protein concentrates and isolates to inactivate aflatoxins. *J. Am. Oil Chem. Soc.* **54**:245A–249A, 1977.
48. Fink, F., Buchner, A., Tiefenbacher, H., Witting, R., and Kohler, W. Decomposition of aflatoxins of feeds. *German Patent #2,517,033*, Nov. 4, 1976.
49. Codifer, L. P. Jr., Mann, G. E., and Dollear, F. G. Aflatoxin inactivation: treatment of peanut meal with formaldehyde and calcium hydroxide. *J. Am. Oil Chem. Soc.* **53**:204–206, 1976.
50. Ciegler, A., Lillehoj, E. B., Peterson, R. E., and Hall, H. H. Microbial detoxification of aflatoxin. *Appl. Microbiol.* **14**:934–939, 1966.
51. Hanssen, E. Aflatoxins. *Med. Ernaehr.* **12**:249–259, 1971.
52. Mann, R. and Rehm, H. J. Degradation of aflatoxin B_1 by microorganisms. *Naturwissenschaften* **62**:537–538, 1975.
53. Ciegler, A., Peterson, R. E., Lagoda, A. A., and Hall, H. H. Aflatoxin production and degradation by *Aspergillus flavus* in 20-liter fermentors. *Appl. Microbiol.* **14**:826–833, 1966.
54. Teunisson, D. J. and Robertson, J. A. Degradation of pure aflatoxins by *Tetrahymena pyriformis. Appl. Microbiol.* **15**:1099–1103, 1967.
55. Arai, T., Ito, T., and Koyama, Y. Antimicrobial activity of aflatoxins. *J. Bacteriol.* **93**:59–64, 1967.
56. Detroy, R. W. and Hesseltine, C. W. Isolation and biological activity of a microbial conversion product of aflatoxin B_1. *Nature* **219**:967, 1968.
57. Cole, R. J., Kirksey, J. W., and Blankenship, B. R. Conversion of aflatoxin B_1 to isomeric hydroxy compounds by *Rhizopus* spp. *J. Agric. Food Chem.* **20**:1100–1102, 1972.
58. Cole, R. J. and Kirksey, J. W. Aflatoxin G_1 metabolism by *Rhizopus* species. *J. Agric. Food Chem.* **19**:222–223, 1971.
59. Lafont, P. and Lafont, J. Metabolism of aflatoxin B_1 by *Aspergillus candidus* Link. *Ann. Microbiol.* **125B**:451–457, 1974.
60. Detroy, R. W. and Hesseltine, C. W. Aflatoxicol: structure of a new transformation product of aflatoxin B_1. *Can. J. Biochem.* **48**:830–832, 1970.

61. Detroy, R. W. and Hesseltine, C. W. Transformation of aflatoxin B_1 by steroid-hydroxylating fungi. *Can. J. Microbiol.* 15:495–500, 1969.
62. Shih, C.-N. and Marth, E. H. Aflatoxin can be degraded by the mycelium of *Aspergillus parasiticus. Z. Lebensm. Unters.-Forsch.* 158:361–362, 1975.
63. Stawicki, S. and Pawlak, J. Microbiological detoxification of aflatoxin B_1. *Poznan. Tow. Przyj. Nauk. Pr. Kom. Nauk. Roln. Kom. Nauk. Les.* 35:307–315, 1973.
64. Dam, R., Tam, S. W., and Satterlee, L. D. Destruction of aflatoxins during fermentation and by-product isolation from artificially contaminated grains. *Cereal Chem.* 54:705–712, 1977.
65. Mann, R. and Rehm, H. J. Degradation products from aflatoxin B_1 by *Corynebacterium rubrum, Aspergillus niger, Trichoderma viride* and *Mucor ambiguus. Eur. J. Appl. Microbiol.* 2:297–306, 1976.
66. Coomes, T. J., Crowther, P. C., Feuell, A. J., and Francis, B. J. Experimental detoxification of groundnut meals containing aflatoxin. *Nature* 209:406–407, 1966.
67. Nabney, J. and Nesbitt, B. F. A spectrophotometric method for determining the aflatoxins. *Analyst* 90:155–160, 1965.
68. Stoloff, L., Trucksess, M., Hardin, N., Francis, O. J., Hayes, J. R., Polan, C. E., and Campbell, T. L. Stability of aflatoxin M in milk. *J. Dairy Sci.* 58:1789–1793, 1975.
69. Mann, G. E., Codifer, L. P. Jr., and Dollear, F. G. Effect of heat on aflatoxins in oilseed meals. *J. Agric. Food Chem.* 15:1090–1092, 1967.
70. Peers, F. G. and Linsell, C. A. Aflatoxin contamination and its heat stability in Indian cooking oils. *Trop. Sci.* 17:229–232, 1975.
71. Fischbach, H. and Campbell, A. D. Note on detoxification of the aflatoxins. *J. Assoc. Off. Agric. Chem.* 48:28, 1965.
72. Dollear, F. G. Detoxification of aflatoxins in foods and feeds. In: *Aflatoxin: Scientific Background, Control and Implications:* 367–371 and 378–384. Goldblatt, L. A. (Ed.). Academic Press, New York, 1969.
73. Quaglia, G. B. Fungal contamination of the food chain. *Boll. Chim. Unione Ital. Lab. Provinciali* 1:74–86, 1975.
74. Lancillotti, F. and Lucisano, A. The aflatoxins. *Ind. Conserve* 46:111–123, 1971.
75. Janicki, J., Szebiotko, K., Chelkowski, J., Kokorniak, M., and Wiewiorowska, M. Aflatoxins in foodstuffs. *Die Nahrung* 16:85–89, 1972.
76. Goldblatt, L. A. Control and removal of aflatoxin. *J. Am. Oil Chem. Soc.* 48:605–610, 1971.
77. *Int. Agency Res. Cancer Monogr.* 1:145, Lyon, France, 1972.
78. Wogan, G. N. Chemical nature and biological effects of the aflatoxins. *Bacteriol. Rev.* 30:460–470, 1966.
79. Jordy, A. Mycotoxin detoxification. *German Patent #2,557,599,* July 7, 1977.

80. Goldblatt, L. A. and Dollear, F. G. Review of prevention, elimination, and detoxification of aflatoxins. *Pure Appl. Chem.* **49**:1759–1764, 1977.

81. Gorst-Allman, C. P., Steyn, P. S., and Wessels, P. L. Oxidiation of the bis-dihydrofuran moieties of aflatoxin B_1 and sterigmatocystin; conformation of tetrahydrofurobenzofurans. *J. Chem. Soc., Perkin Trans.* **1**:1360–1364, 1977.

82. Swenson, D. H., Miller, J. A., and Miller, E. C. The reactivity and carcinogenicity of aflatoxin B_1-2,3-dichloride, a model for the putative 2,3-oxide metabolite of aflatoxin B_1. *Cancer Res.* **35**:3811–3823, 1975.

83. Viroben, G., Delort-Laval, J., Colin, J., and Adrian, J. Aflatoxin inactivation after ammonia treatment. *In vitro* studies on detoxified peanut meals. *Ann. Nutr. Aliment.* **32**:167–185, 1978.

84. Doyle, M. P. and Marth, E. H. Aflatoxin is degraded by fragmented and intact mycelia of *Aspergillus parasiticus* grown 5 to 18 days with and without agitation. *J. Food Prot.* **41**:549–555, 1978.

85. Doyle, M. P. and Marth, E. H. Aflatoxin at several initial concentrations is degraded by different amounts of mycelium of *Aspergillus parasiticus*. *Z. Lebensm. Unters.-Forsch.* **166**:359–362, 1978.

GENERAL

GENERAL PROCEDURES

Degradation Technique	Remarks	Reference
Chemical	A comprehensive text on chemical mutagens, including their chemical reactivities, which may be of use in developing degradation procedures.	1
Chemical	A review discussing the degradation of organo-chlorine insecticides by chemical procedures and comparing the products with those formed during metabolism.	2
Chemical Physical	A review (447 references) giving various procedures and class reactions that can be used to alter organic compounds before GLC analysis.	3
Chemical Physical	A practical guide for removing pollutants from air and water; based mainly on information available in patent literature.	4
Chemical Physical Microbial	A review (701 references) of the toxicity, methods for analysis, and decontamination of specific organic pollutants in water supplies.	5
Chemical Microbial	A review (42 references) on the removal of organic pollutants, including pesticides and polychlorinated biphenyls, from wastewater.	6
Microbial	Bacteria from a sewage lagoon were used for testing the biodegradability of chlorinated and phosphorylated insecticides.	7
Microbial	Bacterial mutants were selected for decomposing organic pollutants in wastewater.	8
Microbial	Bacterial episomal transfer factors were implicated in developing strains capable of degrading resistant organic compounds.	9
Microbial	A review (150 references) on the metabolism of aromatic compounds and the regulation of the pathways involved.	10

GENERAL PROCEDURES
(continued)

Degradation Technique	Remarks	Reference
Microbial	A review (182 references) on the metabolism of hydrocarbons. About 100 species of micro-organisms were able to attack hydrocarbons, especially when emulsified or dispersed by adsorption on inert solids.	11
Microbial	Some organic compounds in wastewater were relatively easily decomposed by activated sludge.	12
Microbial	The addition of mutant bacteria to activated sludge was mentioned in this paper, which briefly described various methods for removing organic chlorides from wastewater.	13
Microbial Oxidation	Twenty pesticides were included in tests of microbial degradation and incineration at $900°C$; no definitive proposals were made.	14
Oxidation	Treatment with chromic acid or heating with 18 M H_2SO_4 with the subsequent addition of HNO_3, if required, degraded most organic compounds. Nitro, azo, and peroxy compounds must be reduced before treatment with the above reagents. Efficient incineration (without loss of toxic volatiles) was recommended when wet oxidation was not feasible.	15
Oxidation	Organic residues, including pesticides, were destroyed in air or wastewater by treatment with $KMnO_4$.	16
Oxidation	The use of a special bomb with HNO_3 at $140°C$ for 2 hr was effective in destroying organic compounds in preparation for trace element analysis.	17
Oxidation	Wet and dry oxidation procedures were described for destroying organic matter. Hazards were noted.	18
Oxidation	Spills of solid carcinogens were wiped up with methanol or dilute methanolic HCl and the	19

GENERAL PROCEDURES
(continued)

Degradation Technique	Remarks	Reference
	washings were treated with dilute aqueous $KMnO_4$ before disposal.	
Oxidation	The detection and removal of peroxides from various compounds (including dioxane and vinyl chloride) were discussed in order to minimize explosion hazards.	20
Oxidation	Toxic organic chemicals of various kinds were removed from wastewater by adsorption on granular activated carbon. The carbon was re-activated by heating at 1600–1800°F with a suitable afterburner and/or air scrubber.	21
Oxidation	Ordinary furnaces were not adequate for the incineration of toxic liquid wastes. A cyclone-apparatus gave good results.	22
Oxidation	An Al-Pt catalyst at 400°C was used to decontaminate air polluted with gaseous products from the thermal decomposition of coal tar pitch (including benzo(a)pyrene).	23
Oxidation	Cl_2 and HCl were recovered during the oxidation of chlorinated organic compounds at less than 450°C in the presence of a Cr catalyst.	24
Oxidation	A highly efficient destruction of hazardous organic materials occurred at 800–1000°C in a furnace containing a molten mixture of 90% Na_2CO_3 and 10% Na_2SO_4.	25
Oxidation	Pesticides and polychlorinated biphenyls were destroyed by incineration with sewage sludge in multiple-hearth furnaces.	26
Oxidation	Use of a liquid injection incinerator and rotary kiln effectively destroyed chemical wastes.	27
Oxidation	Use of a fluidized-bed incinerator effectively destroyed certain chemical wastes.	28

GENERAL PROCEDURES
(continued)

Degradation Technique	Remarks	Reference
Oxidation	The use of ships for at-sea incineration of organochlorine waste products was described; 2400–2700°F temperatures were recommended, with a residence time of 0.5–1.5 sec.	29
Oxidation	Incineration at about 1350°C was used for destroying chlorinated hydrocarbons on ships at sea.	30
Oxidation Chemical	Twenty pesticides were studied. Incineration was found to be superior to chemical procedures for the destruction of waste pesticides.	31
Oxidation Microbial	Industrial wastewater can be effectively detoxified by use of a two-step process: wet air oxidation at 350–610°F, followed by aeration of activated sludge containing activated carbon.	32
Oxidation Ionizing radiation	A commercial system for destroying organic chemicals and microorganisms by air-oxidation and gamma radiation with ^{60}Co was described.	33
Ionizing radiation	Gamma radiation was used for degrading pesticides and other pollutants in water.	34
Ozonation	A commercial procedure was developed for the decolorization of dyes in wastewater by treatment with O_3.	35
Ozonation	O_3 treatment was studied for the disinfection as well as the oxidation of organic pollutants in industrial-municipal wastewater.	36
Ozonation	Ozonation may be an effective method for inactivating carcinogens in water, as judged by the Ames mutagenesis assay.	37
Ozonation Photo-decomposition	A commercial system is available for destroying organic chemicals in water by treatment with O_3 and UV light.	38

GENERAL PROCEDURES
(continued)

Degradation Technique	Remarks	Reference
Ozonation Photo- decomposition	Chlorinated compounds in wastewater were oxidized with O_3 or by O_3 plus UV treatment.	39
Photo- decomposition	A review, with 102 references, discussing the factors involved in the decomposition of herbicides by UV and sunlight.	40
Photo- decomposition	Organic compounds were destroyed by high-energy laser flashes of relatively long duration. C and Cl_2 were among the products produced from CCl_4. The reaction can be violent.	41
Photo- decomposition Microbial Hydrolysis	The fate of organic pesticides in the aquatic environment was discussed. Also included information on adsorption.	42
Photo- decomposition Microbial Chemical	A review of mechanisms for degrading hazardous materials, with emphasis on pesticides. A suggested technology for detoxifying wastes was presented in general terms.	43
Reduction	Chlorinated compounds in wastewater were reduced by Fe powder and a catalyst in a commercial system.	44
Thermal	"Mild" heating, below combustion temperature, was effective in partially degrading 12 pesticides by processes such as dehalogenation and decarboxylation.	45
Thermal	The theory and apparatus for very low pressure pyrolysis were described and applied to kinetic studies of volatile organic compounds.	46
Thermal	The theory and apparatus for the very low pressure pyrolysis were further described. The method was used to study the mechanisms of decomposition of propyl iodides.	47
Chlorination	Toxic organochlorine compounds were further chlorinated in a vapor phase reaction to give	48

GENERAL PROCEDURES
(continued)

Degradation Technique	Remarks	Reference
	CCl_4, HCl and $COCl_2$ as products, which could be of commercial value.	
Reaction with Na biphenyl reagent Reaction with metallic Na (or Li) and liquid NH_3 Oxidation	Nineteen pesticides were degraded by various procedures. The Na-liquid NH_3 treatment was very efficient, but dangerous to use, and the product toxicity was not determined.	49
Exposure to cell culture medium	The Ames mutagen assay was used to determine the biologic $T_{1/2}$ of a variety of direct-acting carcinogens during exposure to cell culture medium at pH 7.2–7.4, 37°C.	50
	Chlorinated pesticides and other hydrophobic organic compounds in wastewater were adsorbed on Amberlite XAD-4. The adsorbent was regenerated with acetone or isopropanol and the pesticides were recovered.	51
	Amberlites were used as adsorbing agents for organic chemicals in wastewater. The pollutants were recovered when the adsorbents were regenerated.	52
	A distillation apparatus was used for removing steam-volatile compounds from water, sediment, and tissue samples. Chemicals were concentrated in a small volume of organic solvent for GLC, but might also be in a convenient form for degradation.	53
	A review of industrial carcinogens and mutagens with numerous references, many of which include metabolic pathways; a few give methods of degradation.	54
Microwave discharge	The rapid and efficient decomposition of methylphosphonates in a small laboratory	55

GENERAL PROCEDURES
(continued)

Degradation Techinque	Remarks	Reference
	reactor indicated that the method holds promise for the destruction of other toxic chemicals in large-volume plasma systems.	
Microwave discharge	Atomic O and free electrons in a reduced pressure plasma resulted in practically complete degradation and oxidation of pesticides and other hazardous wastes. No toxic by-products were formed which could not be treated with caustic.	56
Oxidation Thermal	A detailed (156 pp.) description of various incineration processes for the disposal of hazardous waste materials. A brief discussion of the pyrolytic conversion of hazardous wastes into useful by-products.	57
Oxidation	Pesticides and their containers were oxidized by air in molten Na_2CO_3 at 800–1000°C. HCl and SO_2 were absorbed by the alkali; only CO_2 and water vapor were discharged into the atmosphere.	58
Dechlorination	Ni_2B was used to catalyze the dechlorination of DDT. The reaction was more effective in methanol than in ethanol or 2-propanol. Sequential treatments, after dehydrating the products, resulted in further dechlorinations. Other organochlorine pesticides have been similarly degraded.	59–62
Physico-chemical	Various commercial systems for adsorbing or degrading toxic chemicals in wastewater were discussed in very general terms, including ion exchange, ultrafiltration, adsorption on activated carbon and organic polymers, incineration, and oxidation by O_3, H_2O_2, Cl_2, NaOCl, or $KMnO_4$. No references.	63
Microbial	A study of the biodegradation of organic compounds that may pollute aquatic systems. Enrichment cultures were developed from	64

GENERAL PROCEDURES
(continued)

Degradation Technique	Remarks	Reference
	natural water sources; $T_{1/2}$ determined for several compounds, but no degradation of benzo(a)pyrene or benz(a)anthracene was detected.	
	A protocol was developed for the quantitative removal of primary aromatic amines from contaminated surfaces: 1) use of a special vacuum cleaner; 2) formation of water-soluble salts of HCl; and 3) formation of methanol-soluble Schiff bases to remove any residual amines. Detailed descriptions of procedures and safety equipment were included. The resulting solutions were discarded in polyethylene bags according to published methods. Removal from painted and stainless steel surfaces was much more effective than from concrete.	65
	Chromogenic and fluorogenic derivatives of primary aromatic amines, 4-nitrobiphenyl, and 4-dimethylaminoazobenzene were used for the detection of nanogram amounts of these chemicals on alcohol-moistened filter paper swipes from contaminated surfaces.	66
Oxidation Photo- decomposition Hydrolysis	A review with 108 references. Data from the author's laboratory were included in the discussion of nonbiological degradation of pesticides and other organic chemicals. The need for complete degradation of pollutants during the treatment of potable water was emphasized in order to avoid the formation of products more harmful than the parent compounds.	67
Physical Chemical	A description was given of the Environmental Protection Agency's Hazardous Spills Treatment Trailer for water. Research and development efforts in the areas of spill prevention and detoxification were also discussed.	68

General Procedures

1. Fishbein, L., Flamm, W. G., and Falk, H. L. *Chemical Mutagens.* Academic Press, New York, 1970.
2. Brooks, G. T. Degradation of organochlorine insecticides; problems and possibilities. In: *Fate of Pesticides in the Environment, IUPAC Int. Congr. Pestic. Chem., 2nd, 1971:* 223–236, Tahori, A. S. (Ed.). Gordon and Breach, New York, 1972.
3. Beroza, M. and Coad, R. A. Reaction gas chromatography. *J. Gas Chromatogr.* 4:199–216, 1966.
4. Sittig, M. *How to Remove Pollutants and Toxic Materials from Air and Water. A Practical Guide.* Noyes Data Corp., Park Ridge, New Jersey, 1977.
5. Suffet, I. H., Friant, S., Marcinkiewicz, C., McGuire, M. J., and Wong, D. T.-L. Organics. *J. Water Pollut. Control Fed.* 47:1169–1241, 1975.
6. Paulson, E. G. How to get rid of toxic organics. *Chem. Eng.* 84(22):21–27, 1977.
7. Halvorson, H., Ishaque, M., Solomon, J., and Grussendorf, O. W. A biodegradability test for insecticides. *Can. J. Microbiol.* 17:585–591, 1971.
8. Sorokulova, I. B. Selection of bacteria with improved decomposing activity using mutagenic factors. In: *Mikrobiol. Metody Bor'by Zagryas. Okruzhayushchei Sredy, Tezisy Dokl. Konf.: Akad. Nauk. SSSR, Nauchn, Tsentr. Biol. Issled.:* 38–40, Lambina, V. A. and Uarova, V. N. (Eds.). Puschino, U.S.S.R., 1975.
9. Waid, J. S. The possible importance of transfer factors in the bacterial degradation of herbicides in natural ecosystems. In: *Residue Reviews* 44:65–71, Gunther, F. A. and Gunther J. D. (Eds.). Springer-Verlag, New York, 1972.
10. Ribbons, D. W. The microbiological degradation of aromatic compounds. *Annu. Rep. Prog. Chem.* 62:445–468, 1965.
11. ZoBell, C. E. Action of microorganisms on hydrocarbons. *Bacteriol. Rev.* 10:1–49, 1946.
12. Matsui, S., Murakami, T., Sasaki, T., Hirose, Y., and Iguma, Y. Activated sludge degradability of organic substances in the waste water of the Kashima Petroleum and Petrochemical Industrial Complex in Japan. *Prog. Water Technol.* 7:645–659, 1975.
13. Nathan, M. F. Choosing a process for chloride removal. *Chem. Eng.* 85(3): 93–100, 1978.
14. Stojanovic, B. J., Kennedy, M. V., and Shuman, F. L. Jr. Edaphic aspects of the disposal of unused pesticides, pesticide wastes, and pesticide containers. *J. Environ. Qual.* 1:54–62, 1972.
15. Craig, N. R. Jr. Disposal of carcinogens and highly toxic chemicals. *Saf. Newsl.* Research and Development Section, National Safety Council. Chicago, Illinois, May 1976.

16. Anderson, C. E. Potassium permanganate control of certain organic residues in air and wastewater. In: *Prog. Hazard Chem. Handl. Disposal, Proc. Symp., 3rd, 1972:* 177–186, Howe, R. H. L. (Ed.). Noyes Data Corp., Park Ridge, New Jersey.

17. Fricke, F. L., Rose, O. Jr., and Caruso, J. A. Microwave-induced plasma coupled to a tantalum-strip vaporization assembly for trace element analysis. *Talanta* 23:317–320, 1976.

18. Gorsuch, T. T. *The Destruction of Organic Matter, Int. Ser. of Monogr. in Anal. Chem. Vol.* 39, Belcher, R. and Frieser, H. (Eds.). Pergamon Press, New York, 1970.

19. Rappaport, S. M. and Campbell, E. E. The interpretation and application of OSHA carcinogen standards for laboratory operations. *J. Am. Ind. Hyg. Assoc.* 37:690–696, 1976.

20. Jackson, H. L., McCormack, W. B., Rondestvedt, C. S., Smeltz, K. C., and Viele, I. E. Control of peroxidizable compounds. *J. Chem. Educ.* 47:175–188, 1970.

21. Hager, D. G. and Rizzo, J. L. Removal of toxic organics from wastewater by adsorption with granular activated carbon. *Chem. Eng. Prog.* 72:57–60, 1976.

22. Baikovskii, V. V. Hygienic characteristics of a method of fire detoxification for liquid industrial wastes. *Gig. Sanit.* 39(12):88–89, 1974.

23. Abaseev, V. K., Lebedev, M. A., Andreeva, G. S., Shaposhnikov, Yu. K., and Kvasov, A. A. Catalytic cleaning of gaseous products secondary to thermal decomposition of coal tar pitch. *Gig. Tr. Prof. Zabol.* 19:12–14, 1975.

24. Johnston, E. L. Low temperature catalytic oxidation of chlorinated compounds to recover chlorine values using chromium-impregnated supported catalysts. *U.S. Patent #3,989,807,* Nov. 2, 1976.

25. Anon. Molten salt decomposes pesticide wastes. *Chem. Eng. News* 55(37): 44, 1977.

26. Anon. Sludge incineration. *Environ. Sci. Technol.* 10:1080–1082, 1976.

27. Clausen, J. F., Johnson, R. J., and Zee, C. A. *Destroying Chemical Wastes in Commercial Scale Incinerators.* Facility Report Number 1—The Marquardt Company. U.S. NTIS PB Rep. 265541, 125 pp., Springfield, Virginia, 1977.

28. Ackerman, D. G., Clausen, J. F., Johnson, R. J., and Zee, C. A. *Destroying Chemical Wastes in Commercial Scale Incinerators.* Facility Report Number 3—Systems Technology. U.S. NTIS PB Rep. 265540, 98 pp., Springfield, Virginia, 1977.

29. Ricci, L. J. Offshore incineration gets limited U.S. backing. *Chem. Eng.* 83(1):86–87, 1976.

30. Miller, S. S. How hot is ocean incineration? *Environ. Sci. Technol.* 9:412–413, 1975.

31. Kennedy, M. V., Stojanovic, B. J., and Shuman, F. L. Jr. Chemical and thermal methods for disposal of pesticides. In: *Residue Reviews* 29:89–104,

Gunther, F. A. and Gunther, J. D. (Eds.). Springer-Verlag, New York, 1969.

32. Wilhelmi, A. R. and Ely, R. B. The treatment of toxic industrial wastewaters by a two-step process. In: *30th Purdue Industrial Waste Conference, 1975:* 288-295.

33. Kohn, P. M. Water treatment system cuts organics. *Chem. Eng.* **84**(17): 108-109, 1977.

34. Cappadona, C., Guarino, P., Calderaro, E., Petruso, S., and Ardica, S. Possible use of high-level radiation for the degradation of some substances present in urban and industrial waters. In: *Radiat. Clean Environ., Proc. Int. Symp., 1975:* 265-284. IAEA, Vienna, Austria.

35. Ikehata, A. Dye works wastewater decolorization treatment using ozone. In: *First International Symposium on Ozone for Water and Wastewater Treatment:* 688-711, Rice, R. G., and Browning, M. E. (Eds.). Int. Ozone Inst., Waterbury, Connecticut, 1975.

36. Nebel, C., Gottschling, R. D., Hutchinson, R. L., McBride, T. J., Taylor, D. M., Pavoni, J. L., Tittlebaum, M. E., Spencer, H. E., and Fleischman, M. Ozone disinfection of industrial-municipal secondary effluents. *J. Water Pollut. Control Fed.* **45**:2493-2507, 1973.

37. Caulfield, M. J. and Burleson, G. R. Inactivation of carcinogens by ozonation as monitored by the Ames mutagenesis assay. *Fed. Proc., Fed. Am. Soc. Exp. Biol.* **36**:1079, 1977.

38. Anon. Ultraviolet light enhances ozonation of organics dissolved in wastewater. *Chem. Eng.* **84**(16):18, 1977.

39. Prengle, H. W. Jr., Mauk, C. E., and Payne, J. E. Ozone/UV oxidation of chlorinated compounds in water. In: *Proc.—Forum Ozone Disinfectant, 1976:* 286-295, Fochtman, E. G., Rice, R. G., and Browning, M. E. (Eds.). Int. Ozone Inst., Syracuse, New York, 1977.

40. Crosby, D. G. and Li, M.-Y. Herbicide photodecomposition. In: *Degradation of Herbicides:* 321-363, Kearney, P. C. and Kaufman, D. D. (Eds.). Marcel Dekker, New York, 1969.

41. Gans, F., Troyanowsky, C., and Valat, P. A new reaction: the photobreakdown of organic compounds by electron cascades. *J. Photochem.* **5**:135-150, 1976.

42. Gould, R. F. (Ed.). *Fate of Organic Pesticides in the Aquatic Environment.* Adv. Chem. Ser. **111**, Am. Chem. Soc., Washington, D.C., 1972.

43. Rogers, C. J. and Landreth, R. L. *Degradation Mechanisms: Controlling the Bioaccumulation of Hazardous Materials.* U.S. NTIS PB Rep. **240748**, 13 pp., Springfield, Virgina, 1975.

44. Anon. Process gobbles up chlorinated compounds. *Chem. Eng.* **83**(17): 51-52, 1976.

45. Stojanovic, B. J., Hutto, F., Kennedy, M. V., and Shuman, F. L. Jr. Mild thermal degradation of pesticides. *J. Environ. Qual.* **1**:397-401, 1972.

46. Benson, S. W. and Spokes, G. N. Very low-pressure pyrolysis. I. Kinetic studies of homogeneous reactions at the molecular level. *J. Am. Chem. Soc.* **89**:2525–2532, 1967.
47. King, K. D., Golden, D. M., Spokes, G. N., and Benson, S. W. Very low-pressure pyrolysis. IV. The decomposition of *i*-propyl iodide and *n*-propyl iodide. *Int. J. Chem. Kinet.* **3**:411–426, 1971.
48. Miller, S. S. Emerging technology of chlorinolysis. *Environ. Sci. Technol.* **8**:18–19, 1974.
49. Kennedy, M. V., Stojanovic, B. J., and Shuman, F. L. Jr. Chemical and thermal aspects of pesticide disposal. *J. Environ. Qual.* **1**:63–65, 1972.
50. Jensen, E. M., LaPolla, R. J., Kirby, P. E., and Haworth, S. R. *In vitro* studies of chemical mutagens and carcinogens. I. Stability studies in cell culture medium. *J. Natl. Cancer Inst.* **59**:941–944, 1977.
51. Kennedy, D. C. Treatment of effluent from manufacture of chlorinated pesticides with a synthetic, polymeric adsorbent, Amberlite XAD-4. *Environ. Sci. Technol.* **7**:138–141, 1973.
52. Simpson, R. M. Separation of organic chemicals from water. In: *Progr. Hazard. Chem. Handl. Disposal, Proc. Symp., 3rd, 1972:* 77–102, Howe, R. H. L. (Ed.). Noyes Data Corp., Park Ridge, New Jersey.
53. Veith, G. D. and Kiwus, L. M. An exhaustive steam-distillation and solvent-extraction unit for pesticides and industrial chemicals. *Bull. Environ. Contam. Toxicol.* **17**:631–636, 1977.
54. Fishbein, L. *Potential Industrial Carcinogens and Mutagens.* Environ. Prot. Agency. (U.S.), EPA **560/5-77-005**, Washington, D. C., 1977.
55. Bailin, L. J., Sibert, M. E., Jonas, L. A., and Bell, A. T. Microwave decomposition of toxic vapor simulants. *Environ. Sci. Technol.* **9**:254–258, 1975.
56. Bailin, L. J., Hertzler, B. L., and Oberacker, D. A. Development of microwave plasma detoxification process for hazardous wastes—Part 1. *Environ. Sci. Technol.* **12**:673–679, 1978.
57. Ottinger, R. S., Blumenthal, J. L., Dal Porto, D. F., Gruber, G. I., Santy, M. J., and Shih, C. C. *Recommended Methods of Reduction, Neutralization, Recovery or Disposal of Hazardous Waste, Vol. III. Disposal process descriptions, ultimate disposal, incineration, and pyrolysis processes.* U.S. NTIS PB Rep. 224582, 248 pp., Springfield, Virginia, 1973.
58. Yosim, S. J., Barclay, K. M., and Grantham, L. F. Destruction of pesticides and pesticide containers by molten salt combustion. *Abstr. Pap., 174th ACS Meeting, Div. Pest. Chem.,* Paper #35, 1977.
59. Dennis, W. H. Jr. and Cooper, W. J. Catalytic dechlorination of organochlorine compounds. I. DDT. *Bull. Environ. Contam. Toxicol.* **14**:738–744, 1975.
60. Dennis, W. H. Jr. and Cooper, W. J. Catalytic dechlorination of organochlorine compounds. II. Heptachlor and chlordane. *Bull. Environ. Contam. Toxicol.* **16**:425–430, 1976.

61. Dennis, W. H. Jr. and Cooper, W. J. Catalytic dechlorination of organo-chlorine compounds. III. Lindane. *Bull. Environ. Contam. Toxicol.* **18**: 57–59, 1977.
62. Cooper, W. J. and Dennis, W. H. Jr. Catalytic dechlorination of organo-chlorine compounds. IV. Mass spectral identification of DDT and hepta-chlor products. *Chemosphere* **7**:299–305, 1978.
63. Metzner, A. V. Target: toxin removal. *Environ. Sci. Technol.* **12**:530–533, 1978.
64. Bohonos, N., Chow, T.-W., and Spanggord, R. J. Some observations on bio-degradation of pollutants in aquatic systems. *Jpn. J. Antibiot.* **30**(Supple-ment):S–275-S–285, 1977.
65. Weeks, R. W. Jr. and Dean, B. J. Decontamination of aromatic amine cancer-suspect agents on concrete, metal, or painted surfaces. *J. Am. Ind. Hyg. Assoc.* **39**:758–762, 1978.
66. Weeks, R. W. Jr., Dean, B. J., and Yasuda, S. K. Detection limits of chemical spot tests toward certain carcinogens on metal, painted, and concrete surfaces. *Anal. Chem.* **48**:2227–2233, 1976.
67. Faust, S. D. Chemical mechanisms affecting the fate of organic pollutants in natural aquatic environments. In: *Fate of Pollutants in the Air and Water Environments, Part* **2**: 318–365, Suffet, I. H. (Ed.). *Advances in Environ-mental Science and Technology, Vol.* **8**. John Wiley & Sons, New York, 1977.
68. Lafornara, J. P. Cleanup after spills of toxic substances. *J. Water Pollut. Control Fed.* **50**:617–627, 1978.

CHEMICAL ABSTRACTS SERVICE (CAS) REGISTRY NUMBER INDEX

123-91-1	p-Dioxane	89
134-32-7	1-Naphthylamine	71
140-79-4	1,4-Dinitrosopiperazine	37
151-56-4	Ethylenimine	56
302-01-2	Hydrazine	99
305-03-3	Chlorambucil	111
334-88-3	Diazomethane	137
366-70-1	Procarbazine·HCl	109
540-73-8	1,2-Dimethylhydrazine	98
542-88-1	Bis(chloromethyl)ether	47
614-95-9	N-Nitroso-N-ethylurethane	45
615-53-2	N-Nitroso-N-methylurethane	45
621-64-7	N-Nitrosodipropylamine	37
671-16-9	Procarbazine (free base)	109
684-93-5	N-Nitroso-N-methylurea	43
722-23-6	3'-Methyl-4-aminoazobenzene	141
759-73-9	N-Nitroso-N-ethylurea	42
924-16-3	N-Nitrosodibutylamine	32
1120-71-4	1,3-Propane sultone	130
1162-65-8	Aflatoxin B_1	142
1165-39-5	Aflatoxin G_1	142
1336-36-3	Polychlorinated biphenyls (unspecified structure)	77
1464-53-5	Diepoxybutane (unspecified isomer)	88
2658-24-4	Dimethylethylenimine (2,2-isomer)	55
4239-10-5	Bromoethyl methanesulfonate	128
6098-44-8	N-Acetoxy-2-fluorenylacetamide	51
7220-81-7	Aflatoxin B_2	142
13073-35-3	L-Ethionine	132
14901-08-7	Cycasin	139
24554-26-5	N-[4-(5-Nitro-2-furyl)-2-thiazolyl]formamide	127
24961-39-5	7-Bromomethylbenz(a)anthracene	19

DEGRADATION OF CHEMICAL CARCINOGENS
An Annotated Bibliography

By Milton W. Slein, Ph.D. and Eric B. Sansone, Ph.D.

Safe disposal of carcinogenic substances is rapidly becoming a vital concern of scientists, manufacturers, engineers, and other professionals who may be exposed to toxic organic materials. Here, in easy-to-use tabular format, are degradation and disposal procedures for chemicals identified as potentially carcinogenic by the U.S. Department of Health, Education, and Welfare.

For each chemical or group of chemicals, 68 tabulations indicate the general types of degradative procedures involved and concisely describe the highlights of relevant publications. Degradation hazards and byproduct toxicities are indicated where known, and degradative procedures applicable to many classes of compounds are described in a separate table under General Procedures. Literature citations are presented at the end of each table, and relevant Chemical Abstract Service registry numbers are indexed at the end of the book.

Designed for fast retrieval of information, the volume provides a short descriptive term for each degradation technique, allowing the user to quickly extract needed information. In general, similiar degradation procedures are grouped together in each table. Over 800 references furnish many citations to earlier literature, supplying a broad base for further literature searches.

This unque compilation provides a wealth of useful information in a conveniently organized format. It will be particularly valuable to research chemists and technicians who may be exposed to toxic organic substances, oncologists who are concerned with the etiology of cancer and chemotherapy, manufacturers of organic chemicals, environmental protection specialists, industrial hygienists, and anyone else whose work involves the disposal, decontamination, or degradation of chemical carcinogens.

ABOUT THE AUTHORS

Milton W. Slein, Ph.D., was Project Manager for Laboratory Studies of the Etiology of Cancer of the Digestive System at the Frederick Cancer Research Center. Since his retirement in 1975 he has been involved